Neuropsychological Evaluation of the Spanish Speaker

CRITICAL ISSUES IN NEUROPSYCHOLOGY

Series Editors

Antonio E. Puente
University of North Carolina, Wilmington

Cecil R. Reynolds
Texas A & M University

Current Volumes in this Series

AGING AND NEUROPSYCHOLOGICAL ASSESSMENT
Asenath La Rue

BEHAVIORAL INTERVENTIONS WITH BRAIN-INJURED CHILDREN
A. MacNeil Horton, Jr.

BRAIN MECHANISMS IN PROBLEM SOLVING AND INTELLIGENCE:
A Lesion Survey of the Rat Brain
Robert Thompson, Francis M. Crinella, and Jen Yu

BRAIN ORGANIZATION OF LANGUAGE AND COGNITIVE PROCESSES
Edited by Alfredo Ardila and Feggy Ostrosky-Solis

HANDBOOK OF HEAD TRAUMA: Acute Care to Recovery
Edited by Charles J. Long and Leslie K. Ross

HANDBOOK OF NEUROPSYCHOLOGICAL ASSESSMENT:
A Biopsychosocial Perspective
Edited by Antonio E. Puente and Robert J. McCaffrey

NEUROPSYCHOLOGICAL EVALUATION OF THE SPANISH SPEAKER
Alfredo Ardila, Mónica Rosselli, and Antonio E. Puente

NEUROPSYCHOLOGY, NEUROPSYCHIATRY, AND BEHAVIORAL
NEUROLOGY
Rhawn Joseph

THE NEUROPSYCHOLOGY OF ATTENTION
Ronald A. Cohen

THE NEUROPSYCHOLOGY OF EPILEPSY
Edited by Thomas L. Bennett

A PRACTICAL GUIDE TO HEAD INJURY REHABILITATION: A Focus on
Postacute Residential Treatment
Michael D. Wesolowski and Arnie H. Zencius

A Continuation Order Plan is available for the series. A continuation order will bring delivery of each new volume immediately upon publication. Volumes are billed only upon actual shipment. For further information, please contact the publisher.

Neuropsychological Evaluation of the Spanish Speaker

Alfredo Ardila and Mónica Rosselli
Instituto Colombiano de Neuropsicología
Bogotà, Colombia

and

Antonio E. Puente
University of North Carolina at Wilmington
Wilmington, North Carolina

PLENUM PRESS • NEW YORK AND LONDON

Library of Congress Cataloging-in-Publication Data

Ardila, Alfredo.
  Neuropsychological evaluation of the Spanish speaker / Alfredo
Ardila, Monica Rosselli, and Antonio E. Puente.
       p.   cm. -- (Critical issues in neuropsychology)
  Includes bibliographical references and index.
  ISBN 0-306-44149-7
  1. Neuropsychological tests. 2. Neuropsychological tests--Cross
-cultural studies. 3. Hispanic Amerians--Medical care. 4. Spanish
language.   I. Rosselli, Monica.   II. Puente, Antonio E.
III. Title.   IV. Series.
  [DNLM: 1. Neuropsychological Tests.   BF 176 A676n 1993]
  RC386.6.N48A73 1993
  616.89'075'08961--dc20
  DNLM/DLC
  for Library of Congress   93-37256
                                                               CIP

This book is not intended as a substitute for appropriate education and training in clinical neuropsychology, as outlined in the International Neuropsychological Society/Division 40 (Clinical Neuropsychology) of the American Psychological Association's (APA) education and training guidelines. To determine the definition of a clinical neuropsychologist, consult Division 40 of APA and the National Academy of Neuropsychology. Furthermore, readers should be thoroughly familiar with and adhere to the American Psychological Association Ethical Principles.

ISBN 0-306-44149-7

©1994 Plenum Press, New York
A Division of Plenum Publishing Corporation
233 Spring Street, New York, N.Y. 10013

Printed in the United States of America

Preface

This book is the culmination of a research program conducted in Colombia during the past several years. The fundamental aim of the program was to develop neuropsychological tests for Spanish speakers, especially elderly individuals and those with limited educational attainment. The lack of norms for these populations represents a significant practical problem not only in developing countries but also in more developed countries. For example, norms are usually obtained with middle-class Anglo-Saxon English-speaking populations, often university students, and such norms do not usually include individuals older than 65 years. Furthermore, very few neuropsychological tests have been developed for Spanish speakers; frequently, tests are translated into Spanish (often poor translations at that), but the norms used are still those obtained from English-speaking populations.

This volume summarizes the normative results of this research program. We anticipate that these tests and norms will be particularly useful in the neuropsychological evaluation of Spanish speakers, especially those with limited educational attainment, and the elderly. The United States represents the fifth largest Spanish-speaking country in the world (after Mexico, Spain, Argentina, and Colombia), with over 20 million speakers. It is anticipated that by the year 2025 there will be as many Hispanics in the United States as members of all other ethnic minority groups combined. Further, about 10% of the U. S. population are considered functionally illiterate, with Hispanics representing an unusually large segment. Finally, in the United States there are more than 35 million people older than 65 years of age. Hence while this volume represents an introduction to the neuropsychological assessment of Spanish speakers, it focuses on the elderly and the illiterate. By no means will the issue of understanding brain-

v

injured Hispanics be resolved with this book. However, this contribution, as limited as it may be, is a first step in addressing a critical deficiency in neuropsychology.

Several normative research studies were carried out by the two senior authors during the development of this research program. Four sample sizes were used in obtaining the results presented in this book. In most cases a sample of 180 subjects was divided into three educational groups (0–5, 6–12, and 13 or more years of formal education) at three age ranges (16–30, 31–50, 51–65 years old) for both sexes—thus, a 3 × 3 × 2 design, with 10 subjects per cell. In other cases a larger sample of 360 normal subjects were divided into three educational levels (as before) at five age ranges (55–60, 61–65, 66–70, 71–75, and 76 or more years) for each sex, with 12 subjects in each cell. For the normalization of the Wechsler Memory Scale, 300 subjects were included, matched according to age (20–29, 30–39, 40–49, 50–59, and 60–69 years old), educational level (0–5, 6–12, and more than 12 years of formal education), and sex. Finally, one of the normative research studies used 200 normal subjects from two extreme educational levels (illiterates and professionals) divided into five age ranges (16–25, 26–35, 36–45, 46–55, and 56–65 years) for each sex. In all cases a neurologic and psychiatric screening examination was administered to ensure that mentally or neurologically impaired subjects were excluded from the sample.

Initially, a general review of the influence of cultural and educational factors on neuropsychological assessment is presented. In Chapters 1 through 4, the 19 tests used in our studies are divided into the following four categories and analyzed: (1) orientation and attention, (2) language, (3) memory, and (4) spatial and praxic abilities. In each case, the general background of the test is presented, the test itself is described, and its application is explained. In addition, information on the administration, scoring, and interpretation of test results is presented. Appropriate norms for brain-damaged and non-brain-damaged subjects are included. While some of the tests presented here are found in the classical neuropsychological literature (e.g., the Mini-Mental State Examination, the Boston Diagnostic Aphasia Examination, the Wechsler Memory Scale, and the Rey-Osterrieth Complex Figure), others were specifically prepared by the authors for research and clinical purposes. In Appendix A, the Spanish versions of most of the tests are presented. (For most of these tests the required materials and special devices are minimal and are often provided in this book. Since these language tests are directed to

Spanish speakers, they require a certain level of knowledge of the Spanish language on the part of the examiners.) Appendix B presents percentages, percentiles, and T scores for nine of the analyzed tests, and norms for four different groups: subjects 55–65 years old with five or fewer years of formal education and subjects more than 65 years old with more than five years of formal education. All the norms are from our studies. Our tests include:

"A" Cancellation Test
Spanish Naming Test (adapted)
Spanish Reading and Writing Test
Spanish Repetition Test
Spanish Phonemic Test (adapted)
Spanish Grammar Test
Verbal Fluency Test (adapted)
A Calculation Abilities Test
Verbal Serial Learning Test
Memory for Unfamiliar Faces (adapted)

Other tests were translated or minimally changed.

Acknowledgments

The publication of this book represents the product of numerous years of test development, standardization, and writing. Many individuals in Colombia and the United States assisted in its completion.

We received the support of many individuals in the preparation of some of the tests. Olga Ardila, Maria Victoria López, Catalina Ramírez, and Lissy Sperber collaborated on the Grammar Test for Spanish Speakers. The Spanish Phoneme Discrimination Test was adapted from materials supplied by Raul Avila. In the Calculation Ability Test, an effort to integrate the contributions of different authors in the testing of arithmetic abilities was made. Other people participated in the collection of the data and in the analysis of the results. Our gratitude is extended to José Ricardo Bateman, Luz Esther Bueno, Nubia Cárdenas, Cielo Castro, Aurora de Colorado, María Mercedes Díaz, Elsy Elena Fajardo, Angela Flórez, Orlando Fontecha, Martha Lucía López, Elbers Medellín, Fanny Moreno, Claudia Pilar Navarro, Jorge Ortiz, Martha Patiño, Carolina Bella Paz, Beatriz Penagos, Margarita Ramírez, Patricia Rosas, Janey Sturtz, Hugo Vásquez, and Magda Piedad Vázquez.

The Fundación Universitaria Konrad Lorenz in Bogotá enthusiastically supported this research program. For one of the research projects we received a grant from the Fondo Colombiano de Investigaciones Científicas y Proyectos Especiales "Francisco José de Caldas" (Colciencias). The Miami Institute of Psychology of the Caribbean Center for Advanced Studies, the Instituto Colombiano de Neuropsicología, and the University of North Carolina at Wilmington provided us with further technical and secretarial assistance. We are indebted to Lydia Woodard and Martha Jo Clemmons, who assisted in revising the manuscript and accompanying tables numerous times. Finally, special thanks goes to Eliot Werner, Executive Editor at Plenum Press, for the development and publication of this clinical manual. From the beginning, his support of this project has been unwavering.

As with any book, the final responsibility for its limitations rests with the authors. We trust, however, that such limitations will be shared with us in an effort both to compare research programs and to improve the status of the field of mutual interest.

Contents

Introduction: Neuropsychological Assessment in Different Cultural Contexts

Numerous well-accepted assumptions abound on the measurement of human brain function. For example, it is well understood and accepted that for the accurate assessment of neuropsychological performance one must have both appropriate instruments and well-trained professionals. The assumption behind this premise is fairly simple: If the testing situation is held appropriately constant, then the dependent measure will be correctly measured.

There is a major problem with this assumption that is beyond the scope of the instruments and qualifications of clinical neuropsychologists. It involves the belief that what is measured—namely, brain function—is relatively, if not completely, immune to such variables as language, culture, age, and education. Indeed, outside of a few contributions to neuropsychology from the standpoint of lifespan development (e.g., LaRue, 1992) and the study of language as a separate entity (e.g., Ardila and Ostrosky-Solis, 1988), little is known about the effects these intervening variables might have on brain function.

One explanation for this paucity of information is the assumption that these variables play, at best, a small part in shaping brain functions. For example, Lezak's (1983) now-classic *Neuropsychological Assessment* contains few references on this topic, and no article addresses the matter in the last volume of *Archives of Clinical Neuropsychology*, the official journal of the National Academy of Neuropsychology. Of the over 3,000 articles on neuropsychological assessment published during the 1980s, subject variables (beyond age and education) were the primary focus in less than 20.

An alternative explanation for this lack of information is that the history of neuropsychological assessment is fairly recent and attention has been paid to the most obvious variables. Whereas some (e.g., Faust, 1992) believe that it is still too early to consider clinical neuropsychology a science, most psychologists and almost all neuropsychologists believe that the discipline is sufficiently well developed to at least make some general (if not specific) statements about brain function. What may be missing from the equation is a variable placing the client/patient in a valid ecological context. We believe it is fair to state that variables beyond test instruments and neuropsychologists' qualifications are critical to understanding brain function. Of the many potential variables (e.g., medication, physiological condition, nutrition, sex, culture, ethnicity, education), some of the most important are ethnocultural and educational in nature. To provide support for the hypothesis of ecological context, we offer the present volume as a means of obtaining a clearer understanding of one type of special client/patient—the Spanish speaker.

There are several reasons why we have chosen Spanish speakers. One, all the authors are Hispanic by birth and consider Spanish our native language and the basis for our primary culture. A second reason is that Hispanics represent approximately 10% of the U.S. population, and worldwide there are approximately 500 million Spanish speakers, compared to about 362 million English speakers (World Population Data Sheet, 1986–1990). Further, in the United States alone, Hispanics will come close to constituting the largest ethnic minority group in the United States by the year 2025 (*Statistical Abstract*, 1990). Another reason for choosing this population is that very few studies using Spanish speakers have been published. Hence, clinical neuropsychologists are presently not equipped to deal with an ever-growing segment of the population they serve. Finally, simple translations of North American/English-based tests are often not sufficient, and sometimes altogether inappropriate, for assessment of Spanish speakers.

LANGUAGE

One potential solution to the problem of obtaining accurate neuropsychological assessment of the Spanish speaker would be to use translations of available tests. There are numerous problems with this approach, however; one has to do with the availability of translated tests. As of late 1991, only the Luria-Nebraska and Halstead Neuropsychological Batteries have been translated into Spanish, with most of the translation being completed in Spain. However, the translations were not authorized, no cross-translations were reported (English to Spanish to English), and no normative data were reported (e.g., Dergan, 1987). It may be worthwhile adding that the Chinese, Greek, and Finnish versions of these tests have similar problems (e.g., Donias, Vassi Lopoulou, Golden, & Lovell, 1989; Xu, Gong, & Matthews, 1987). Translations of other tests (e.g., Wechsler Memory Test) have yet to be made widely available.

Phonological and grammatical concerns should also be addressed. The Luria-Nebraska, for example, is heavily language-based and contains two scales devoted to measuring communication abilities. Many of the items assume knowledge of certain culturally based sounds (e.g., s-t-o-n-e, since s and t do not occur together in initial position in Spanish, it makes no sense to test for a "st" sound) or concepts (e.g., proverbs). To simply translate these items would result in an inaccurate measurement because a dependent measure of a culturally (and not neuropsychologically) based variable may be contaminated by ignorance.

OTHER VARIABLES

Besides language, other variables may play a role in the measurement of human brain function (e.g., Badcock & Ross, 1982). While we acknowledge that many other variables are probably critical to understanding brain function (see Puente & McCaffrey, 1992), we stress three, besides age, that we feel play an important role in understanding brain function in Spanish speakers.

Culture is a broadly defined concept referring to a large group that holds general concepts about human behavior. In contrast, ethnicity is often considered to reflect group composition in which membership is based on common descent, physical characteristics, customs, heritage, and concepts. An excellent example of the application of ethnicity to neuropsychology is found in Badcock and Ross's (1982) suggestions on how to test Australian Aborigines. These suggestions focus on changing the testing to accommodate the limitations of the English language and Australian culture in understanding the native Aborigines. With Hispanics, culture-sensitive tests could involve the role of religion and the family in explaining behavior.

Another important and previously poorly understood variable is education. Neuropsychologists have generally accepted the notion that intellectual ability and educational level affect certain types of neuropsychological tests (e.g., the Category Test). However, only the Luria-Nebraska Test uses education to systematically determine brain impairment. Further, the validity of most neuropsychological tests becomes weak when testing individuals with very low educational attainment. For example, Rosselli, Ardila, and Rosas (1990) recently reported that illiterates significantly differed from a matched control on tests assessing phonological discrimination, the ability to name figures, buciofacial praxis, coordinated movements, and cancellation. What is particularly surprising in this study is not that significant differences were found (indeed, they were expected) but that fine visuomotor movements appear to be affected by educational attainment. Thus, the traditional belief that motor functions are immune to psychosocial influence no longer appears to be true.

POTENTIAL SOLUTIONS

Whether one is dealing with Hispanics or any other minority or ethnic group, ecological validity is of major importance. There are several ways of increasing the validity of neuropsychological assessment beyond continuing to improve test instruments and the training of clinical neuropsychologists.

The first approach involves translators. Testing should not proceed with the use of a translator, especially if he or she is a family member. There are many concepts and words that are not common to a nonpsychologist translator; thus, the use of a translator could result in mistranslation of either the question or the response. Objectivity is often questionable as well. Second, tests cannot simply be translated. As indicated earlier, many phonological and cultural variables do not lend themselves to a corresponding translation. Comprehensive knowledge of the Hispanic culture and the Spanish language are essential in conducting a valid assessment of a Spanish-speaking subject. Another issue, and one not addressed in this volume, is that there are many Spanish regional variations. Thus, a test translated and standardized in Spain may not be appropriate for Mexican populations. Specific sensitivity to subcultures is critical.

Another issue of importance is that of normative data. Few

translations report corresponding normative data. The studies that do report norms use small samples and inadequate sampling procedures. To date, no study has been published using norms from Spanish speakers residing in separate countries. Associated with this issue is the question of native versus acquired language: for example, would a native English speaker, fluent in Spanish at the time of testing, perform similarly or equivalently on the English and Spanish versions of a test? The answer to this question may still be years away.

Finally, a case should be made for clinical sensitivity. It is well known that nonmajority status is often associated with poor psychological test performance (Puente, 1990). Besides recognizing the importance of appropriate translations and norms, the clinical neuropsychologist must entertain the notion that human diversity does not translate into human deficiency. Care must be taken to be sensitive to cultural, ethnic, language, and other, diversity in understanding human brain function. To do otherwise coinstitutes a disservice to the field and an ethical violation.

SUMMARY AND FUTURE DIRECTIONS

The current status of clinical neuropsychology suggests unprecedent growth and acceptance within the psychological and health community. This growth, unfortunately, has not encompassed a comprehensive understanding of the patient's context. Of the numerous variables that could be addressed in an effort to increase ecological validity, we have chosen to focus on language, culture, education, and age. This volume presents a translation and partial standardization for several commonly used neuropsychological tests.

While we trust that this contribution to the literature will enhance an appreciation of the patient's context in general, and Hispanics patients in particular, we propose consideration of the following areas in the continuing pursuit of ecological validity in clinical neuropsychological assessment:

1. *Sensitivity*. The clinician as well as the academician (researcher or professor) must be sensitive to the fact that much that is not known about the client/patient is not directly neurological in origin. Caution should be used when testing patients of a different cultural or ethnic background.

2. *Knowledge Base*. Clearly much more research on ecological

validity is needed. However, care must be taken to delineate the appropriate variables in conjunction with methodological rigor.

3. *Specialty.* Neuropsychological training is a relatively new activity within psychology. Indeed, many of those practicing today do not have formal neuropsychological training. However, subspecialties will probably arise even within the field of neuropsychology. We propose that the area of cross-cultural neuropsychology be considered as a separate specialty area.

Chapter 1

Orientation and Attention

MINI–MENTAL STATE EXAMINATION

Background

The Mini–Mental State Examination (MMSE) (Folstein, Folstein, & McHugh, 1975) was developed as a quick and simple cognitive function test. It is divided into six sections: orientation, registration, attention and calculation, recall, language, and constructional. The administration takes from 5 to 10 minutes, and the maximum score is 30 points. The test was initially standardized on 63 normal subjects aged 55 and above. "Elderly" subjects and younger patients with functional psychiatric disorders achieved scores between 25 and 28.

This test has proven useful in recognizing changes in the intellectual functioning of psychiatric and neurological patients (Lezak, 1983), and it is widely used in research with demented patients. It has been found to have adequate interrater reliability, and adequate test–retest reliability (Nelson, Fogel, & Faust, 1986).

Normative Data

A Spanish version (including the figure) of the Folstein and colleagues' Mini–Mental State Examination is found in Appendix A1. Some of the questions have been slightly adjusted to the cultural characteristics of the population studied.

The Spanish version of the MMSE was given to 346 neurologically normal subjects. A brief neurological and psychiatric screening was initially administered to screen for neurological or psychiatric problems. All subjects performed adequately in activities of daily living. Subjects were divided into groups according to age

(55–60, 61–65, 66–70, 71–75, and over 75 years), sex, and educational level (0–5, 6–12, and more than 12 years of formal education). Table 1.1 presents the demographic characteristics of the standardization population.

Normative data are presented in Table 1.2. No differences were found between the sexes. There is a mild tendency to obtain lower scores with increasing age across all three educational groups. Differences between extreme educational groups is approximately three points. The most important decrease in low-education subjects is observed after 65 years, in the higher educational groups after 70 years. For low-education subjects older than 75, the average score is 23.32 points. Usually, the criterion employed to differentiate normal and pathological populations has been 23 points. Note that differences among educational groups are more important than differences among age groups.

Comments

Recently, Bleecker, Bolla-Wilson, Kawas, and Agnew (1988) published a normalization of the MMSE in 194 white, healthy Anglo subjects (87 men, 107 women). Their mean educational level was 14.4 years. They reported scores higher than the scores we found; their results are comparable only to our highest educational group. Despite the fact that they divided their subjects into age groups different from ours and presented their results in terms of medians and not means, their normalization scores are about one to two points higher than those reported here for every age range.

TABLE 1.1. Distribution of the 346 Neurologically
Normal Subjects of the Standardization Sample
According to Age, Education, and Sex

	Age (in years)					
Education	55–60 (M/F)	61–65 (M/F)	66–70 (M/F)	71–75 (M/F)	> 75 (M/F)	Total
0–5 years	12/11	11/10	10/10	9/11	10/12	52/54
6–12 years	12/12	12/12	14/13	11/11	11/12	60/60
> 12 years	13/12	11/12	13/14	11/11	12/11	60/60
Total	37/35	34/34	37/37	31/33	33/35	172/174

TABLE 1.2. Mean Scores for the Mini–Mental
State Examination in 346 Normal Elderly Subjects
by Age and Educational Level

Eduation	Age				
	56–60	61–65	66–70	71–75	< 75
0–5 years	25.06	25.01	23.67	23.55	23.32
6–12 years	28.46	27.88	27.71	25.97	24.60
> 12 years	28.58	28.00	27.88	27.36	25.84

Escobar, Burman, Karno, Forsythe, Landsverk, and Golding (1986) administered the MMSE to samples of the Hispanic and Anglo populations in the Los Angeles area. They found that some of the items were sensitive not only to educational level but also to the cultural background of the subject. The Hispanic group presented a higher number of errors to questions related to the current season and to the concept of state. Seasons are not particularly relevant to orientation in the majority of the tropical and subtropical Spanish-speaking countries (rainy vs. nonrainy may be a more important distinction). State and country can be confusing concepts for anyone not used to those terms: a state is, strictly speaking, a country, not just the division of a country, and, even worse, the name of this country includes the word *state*. Thus, it is not surprising that these two items are sensitive to cultural background. Items found most sensitive to education were those requiring reading, spelling, and math. Six of the items were sensitive to age and eight to educational level. Hence, education was a heavier factor on observed scores than age.

Folstein, Anthony, Parhad, Duffy, and Gruenberg (1985) studied 3,481 elderly adults not living in institutions. They found that only 20% of the 65-and-over population scored under 23 on the MMSE and proposed that this score be considered an adequate cutoff point for distinguishing normal and abnormal aging. In contrast, Bleecker and associates (1988) advised a higher cutoff score.

Kafonek, Ettinger, Roca, Kittner, Taylor, and German (1989) used the MMSE in a long-term care facility. They found it between 81% and 83% sensitive in screening for dementia when using the general cutoff point of 23. In addition, the MMSE was found to be significantly correlated with functional status ($r = .48$). Farber, Schmitt, and

Logue (1988) found a correlation of .83 between MMSE scores and full-scale IQs.

Magaziner, Bassett, and Hebel (1987) observed a significant effect of age and education on the MMSE. Kokmen, Naessens, and Offord (1987) observed a correlation of −.23 between age and total score on the MMSE and .35 between educational level and total score. Their results are in agreement with the present results, namely, that educational level is an even more important variable than age in determining a mental status examination score. Therefore, unless scores are also interpreted according to educational level, age norms would be inaccurate.

"A" CANCELLATION TEST

Background

The "A" Cancellation Test is generally used to assess sustained attention. It consists of a series of random letters or numbers (usually 60 or more) distributed in a paper. The subject is required to cross out one specific letter or number as quickly as possible. Strub and Black (1981) used A as the target letter. This task is easily performed by a person whose sustained attention is intact. Thus, even one or two lapses in this test may reflect an attention problem (Lezak, 1983). Errors included both omission errors, failure to cross out As, and addition errors, crossing out any letter other than A (Strub & Black, 1981).

Normative Data

A matrix of letters with 20 columns and 8 rows was prepared. In the 160 letters the letter A appears 16 times (see Appendix A, Section A2), equally distributed in the right and left halves of the matrix. Subjects were asked to cross out all As fast as possible and following any order.

The test was given to 346 subjects divided into groups according to age (56–60, 61–65, 66–70, 71–75, and over 75 years), sex, and educational level (0–5, 6–12, and more than 12 years of formal education). An analysis of variance disclosed that the influence of sex was not statistically significant, although age ($F = 5.21$; $df = 4$; $p<.0001$) and educational level ($F = 11.56$; $df = 2$; $p<.0001$) were

TABLE 1.3. "A" Cancellation Test Mean Scores
by Age and Educational Level (N = 346)

Education	Age (in years)				
(years)	55–59	60–65	66–70	71–75	> 75
0–5	14.30	13.81	13.65	11.45	13.36
6–12	15.21	15.33	14.59	14.32	12.78
> 12	15.20	15.04	15.30	15.36	13.74
Means	14.90	14.72	14.41	13.71	13.29

statistically significant. Interaction between both variables was also significant ($F = 2.26$; $df = 8$; $p<.02$). Table 1.3 presents the results obtained for different age and educational groups.

Norms (percentages, percentiles, and T scores) were obtained for four groups with the following age and educational level dimensions: 55–65 years old and 0–5 years of formal education; 55–65 years and more than 5 years of formal education; over 65 and 0–5 years of formal education; and over 65 and more than 5 years of formal education (see Appendix B, Table B1).

DIGIT SYMBOL TEST

Background

Digit Symbol is the last subtest of both the original and revised Wechsler Adult Intelligence Scale (WAIS) (Wechsler, 1955, 1985). It is basically a psychomotor ability test, with motor persistence, attention, response speed, and visuomotor coordination playing an important role in the individual's performance.

Digit Symbol consists of a page of four rows of small blank squares (100 in all), each square beneath a number from 1 to 9. Above these rows is a printed key that pairs each number with a different symbol. The first ten squares constitute a practice trial. The subject's task is to fill in the squares with the symbol that is paired to the number in the key. After 90 seconds in adults (or 120 in children), the subject is stopped; the score earned is the correct number of squares filled. This test is particularly difficult for elderly subjects, whose vision or visuomotor coordination is decreased (Savash, Britton, Bolton, & Hall, 1973).

Mean score for children 8 and older is 30–31 (in 120 seconds); for normal children 15 years of age the mean score is 60–63 (Wechsler, 1974). For the Wechsler Adult Intelligence Scale–Revised, the mean score for normal subjects 20–34 years old is 57–61 (in 90 seconds). However, the WAIS-R Manual does not present the raw scores on the Digit Symbol test for elderly subjects. The correction by age is only completed as part of the IQ score. It is important to note that the Digit Symbol test is one of the most sensitive test to effects of aging, accounting for a significant proportion of the decline in neuropsychological performance in elderly subjects (Ardila & Rosselli, 1989).

Normative Data

The Digit Symbol test was administered to 346 subjects divided into groups according to age (56–60, 61–65, 66–70, 71–75, and more than 75 years), sex, and educational level (0–5, 6–12, and more than 12 years of formal education). The administration system described for the WAIS-R (Wechsler, 1985) was used, except that subjects were allowed 120 seconds. Table 1.4 shows the F values for the three variables analyzed. Note that differences are statistically significant for all three variables (age, educational level, and sex). Interaction between age and educational level was also statistically significant.

Performance for this test significantly decreases with age and increases with educational attainment. In general, performance was better for males than for females (Table 1.5) but differences between

TABLE 1.4. F Values in the Digit Symbol Test
Administered the Standardization Sample

	df	Mean square	F	Level of significance
Educational level (A)	2	10578.203	76.796	.001
Age (B)	4	2896.467	21.028	.001
Sex (C)	1	823.560	5.979	.015
A × B	8	370.197	2.688	.007
A × C	2	46.068	0.334	NS
B × C	4	67.078	0.487	NS
A × B × C	8	98.348	0.714	NS

TABLE 1.5. Digit Symbol Mean Scores for Both
Sexes at Various Age Ranges and Educational Levels

Education	56–60	61–65	66–70	71–75	> 75
			Age		
0–5 years					
Male	17.96	17.64	17.45	11.44	9.35
Female	13.86	12.70	10.25	12.27	10.15
Combined	16.00	14.76	13.85	11.90	9.75
6–12 years					
Male	36.00	25.29	22.36	23.41	12.59
Female	28.63	24.75	23.92	17.36	13.33
Combined	32.31	25.02	23.11	20.39	12.98
> 12 years					
Male	45.96	45.00	36.62	34.18	16.75
Female	40.46	33.33	33.54	28.91	14.91
Combined	41.24	38.91	35.02	31.55	15.87
Average					
Male	31.97	28.97	25.47	23.01	12.89
Female	27.65	23.59	22.57	19.51	12.79

the sexes tend to decrease with age, from 4.32 in the first age range
(56–60 years) to 0.10 in the last age range (more than 75 years).

Norms (percentiles and T scores) were obtained for four groups
with the following age and educational level dimensions: 55–65
years old and 0–5 years of formal education; 55–65 years and more
than 5 years of formal education; over 65 and 0–5 years of formal
education; and over 65 and more than 5 years of formal education.
See Appendix B, Table B2.

Results in Brain-Damaged Populations

The Digit Symbol test is the WAIS subtest most sensitive to brain
damage. As a speed, motor, attentional, and perceptual test, it is
particularly sensitive to any type of brain damage, and even minimal
brain damage can affect scores. However, norms for brain-damaged
patients are not available.

Patients with motor disturbances, such as those with Parkinson's
disease and Huntington's disease, do poorly on this test as a result of
either hypo- or hyperkinesia. Motor aphasics usually present right

hemiparesis, with performance with the right hand being impaired while performance with the left hand is not affected. In general, patients with any type of motor dysfunction should not be given this test. Patients with right-hemisphere damage and spatial hemi-neglect encounter specific difficulty in visually exploring the squares on the left side of the test. Patients with frontal lobe damage perseverate and, consequently, will do poorly on this test, as will brain-damaged patients with difficulties in discriminating figures. In cases of left-hemisphere damage, difficulties in understanding the instructions may be evident.

Language

BOSTON DIAGNOSTIC APHASIA EXAMINATION

Background

One of the most widely used tests for diagnosing aphasic language disturbances is the Boston Diagnostic Aphasia Examination (BDAE) (Goodglass & Kaplan, 1972), which was translated into Spanish in 1979 and published in Argentina. In 1980 a normative study of the test using an English-speaking population suggested that the effects of age and educational level were critical in addressing aphasia deficits (Borod, Goodglass, & Kaplan, 1980). In 1983 a second English edition was published (Goodglass & Kaplan, 1983) with a few minor changes made in the test procedure. The scoring system was revised (Z scores were changed to percentiles), and norms for neurologically normal adults were included. In 1986 the second edition was translated into Spanish in Spain; this edition included data obtained from 40 aphasic patients (Garcia-Albea, Sanchez-Bernardos, & del Viso-Pabon, 1986). Rosselli, Ardila, Florez, and Castro (1990) reported on a normalization of the Spanish version of the BDAE while analyzing the influence of age, sex, and educational level on its subtests.

Test Description

The BDAE was developed by Goodglass and Kaplan (1979) to provide more "insight" into the functioning of aphasics and to relate the test scores to standard neurological classification of aphasic disorders. The test contains seven sections, each focusing on one area of expressive speech. The following areas of verbal communication are evaluated: articulation, verbal fluency, word-finding difficulty, repetition, seriatim speech, grammar and syntax, paraphasia, auditory comprehension, reading, and writing. Within each of the sections, several issues are addressed in greater detail. For example, in the section on repetition, the following issues are further considered: repetition of words, high-probability repetition, low-probability repetition, word reading, responsive naming, visual confrontation naming, body-part naming, and animal naming.

Normative Data

Normative data were obtained with 180 neurologically normal native Spanish-speaking subjects, grouped according to age (16–30, 31–50, and 51–65 years), educational level (0–5, 6–12, and more than 12 years of formal education), and sex. The Spanish version of the BDAE prepared by Silvia Cuschnir de Fairman (Goodglass & Kaplan, 1979) was used; the Paraphasias, Music, Articulation Agility, and Verbal Ability sections were not included.

Correlations of age and education with test performance on all 28 subtests was performed. Table 2.1 presents the correlations of age and educational level with test performance on all 28 subtests. Correlations between age and test performance on all subtests except Phrase Length, Commands, Responsive Naming, Body-Part Naming, Word Reading, Repetition of Words, Automatized Sequences, Reciting, Mechanics in Writing, Sentences to Dictation, and Narrative Writing were statistically significant. A significant correlation between educational level and test performance was observed in all subtests, except Commands, Repetition of Words, and Reciting. Thus, education may be more critical in BDAE than age.

Table 2.2 shows the means and standard deviations of the scores for the different subtests. Observe that, in general, increasing age is associated with lower scores and higher standard deviations and that scores are higher for subjects with a higher educational level. For some of the subtests, such as Commands and Repetition of Words, differences between groups are minimal or nonexistent. This is due to the fact that the ceiling was too low to recognize differences within the age ranges included in this study.

TABLE 2.1. Correlations between Age and
Educational Level for Subtests of the Boston
Diagnostic Aphasia Examination (BDAE)

Subtests	Age		Education level	
	r	p	r	p
Fluency				
Phrase Length	.01	NS	.36	.001
Auditory Comprehension				
Word Discrimination	−.20	.003	.36	.001
Body-Part Identification	−.13	.03	.48	.001
Commands	.00	NS	.00	NS
Complex Material	−.17	.01	.47	.001
Naming				
Responsive Naming	−.01	NS	.18	.007
Confrontation	−.24	.001	.50	.001
Animal Naming	−.18	.007	.28	.001
Body-Part Naming	.05	NS	.42	.001
Oral Reading				
Word Reading	−.10	NS	.38	.001
Oral Sentence	−.23	.001	.35	.001
Repetition				
General Words	.00	NS	.00	NS
High-Probability Words	−.28	.001	.26	.001
Low-Probability Words	−.40	.001	.24	.001
Automatic Speech				
Automatized Sequences	−.06	NS	.39	.001
Reciting	.00	NS	.00	NS
Reading Comprehension				
Symbol Discrimination	−.29	.001	.41	.001
Word Recognition	−.21	.003	.32	.001
Oral Spelling	−.44	.001	.57	.001
Word–Picture Matching	−.18	.01	.39	.001
Sentences–Paragraphs	−.26	.001	.59	.001
Writing				
Mechanics	−.11	NS	.36	.001
Serial Writing	−.25	.001	.42	.001
Primer-Level Dictation	−.17	.01	.35	.001
Written Confrontation	−.39	.001	.29	.001
Spelling to Dictation	−.35	.001	.24	.001
Sentences to Dictation	−.12	NS	.44	.001
Narrative Writing	−.11	NS	.64	.001

TABLE 2.2. Means (and Standard Deviations) for Groups of Normal Subjects of Different Ages and Educational Levels on the Boston Diagnostic Aphasia Examination (N = 180)

	Years of education								
	0–5			6–12			13 or more		
	Age								
Subtests	16–30	31–50	51–65	16–30	31–50	51–65	16–30	31–50	51–65
Fluency									
Phrase Length	6.65	6.67	6.77	7.00	7.00	7.00	7.00	7.00	7.00
	(0.78)	(0.77)	(0.68)	(0.00)	(0.00)	(0.00)	(0.00)	(0.00)	(0.00)
Auditory Comprehension									
Word Discrimination	68.00	68.17	62.77	72.00	71.71	68.10	72.00	72.00	71.15
	(6.13)	(6.82)	(18.36)	(0.00)	(1.07)	(5.49)	(0.00)	(0.00)	(2.35)
Body-Part Identification	18.65	19.33	17.73	19.77	19.93	19.50	19.94	20.00	20.00
	(1.61)	(1.24)	(2.55)	(1.06)	(0.24)	(2.54)	(0.23)	(0.00)	(0.00)
Commands	15.00	15.00	15.00	15.00	15.00	15.00	15.00	15.00	15.00
	(0.00)	(0.00)	(0.00)	(0.00)	(0.00)	(0.00)	(0.00)	(0.00)	(0.00)
Complex Material	9.47	9.33	9.18	10.55	11.14	9.80	11.11	11.32	10.90
	(2.03)	(1.91)	(1.92)	(1.71)	(1.23)	(1.10)	(1.23)	(1.07)	(1.02)
Naming									
Responsive Naming	29.70	29.50	29.32	29.86	30.00	30.00	30.00	30.00	30.00
	(0.85)	(2.12)	(2.34)	(0.64)	(0.00)	(0.00)	(0.00)	(0.00)	(0.00)
Confrontation	101.94	101.28	97.54	104.77	105.00	102.00	105.00	105.00	105.00
	(4.16)	(6.18)	(9.24)	(1.06)	(0.00)	(4.70)	(0.00)	(0.00)	(0.00)
Animal Naming	15.29	16.50	14.36	16.77	16.78	15.60	17.50	17.48	16.60
	(2.95)	(3.22)	(3.77)	(2.52)	(2.51)	(3.65)	(1.85)	(2.47)	(2.06)
Body-Part Naming	26.59	20.05	26.68	28.77	29.64	30.00	30.00	30.00	30.00
	(4.18)	(2.48)	(5.18)	(2.79)	(1.33)	(0.00)	(0.00)	(0.00)	(0.00)

Oral Reading									
Word Reading	30.00 (0.00)	30.00 (0.00)	30.00 (0.00)	30.00 (0.00)	30.00 (0.00)	29.95 (0.21)	29.41 (1.80)	26.78 (8.11)	26.14 (7.55)
Oral Sentence	10.00 (0.00)	10.00 (0.00)	10.00 (0.00)	8.50 (0.40)	10.00 (0.00)	10.00 (0.00)	10.00 (0.00)	9.33 (2.38)	8.36 (2.59)
Repetition									
Word	10.00 (0.00)	10.00 (0.00)	10.00 (0.00)	10.00 (0.00)	10.00 (0.00)	10.00 (0.00)	10.00 (0.00)	10.00 (0.00)	10.00 (0.00)
High-Probability	8.00 (0.00)	8.00 (0.00)	8.00 (0.00)	7.90 (0.40)	8.00 (0.00)	8.00 (0.00)	8.00 (0.00)	7.78 (0.65)	7.36 (1.14)
Low-Probability	7.90 (0.40)	8.00 (0.00)	8.00 (0.00)	7.70 (0.80)	8.00 (0.00)	8.00 (0.00)	7.88 (0.48)	7.89 (0.47)	6.36 (2.19)
Automatic Speech									
Automatized Sequences	8.00 (0.00)	8.00 (0.00)	8.00 (0.00)	8.00 (0.00)	7.93 (0.27)	7.95 (0.21)	7.59 (0.79)	7.89 (0.32)	7.45 (0.91)
Reciting	2.00 (0.00)	2.00 (0.00)	2.00 (0.00)	2.00 (0.00)	2.00 (0.00)	2.00 (0.00)	2.00 (0.00)	2.00 (0.00)	2.00 (0.00)
Reading Comprehension									
Symbol Discrimination	9.80 (0.61)	10.00 (0.00)	10.00 (0.00)	9.40 (1.74)	10.00 (0.00)	10.00 (0.00)	9.76 (0.75)	9.61 (1.14)	8.36 (1.91)
Word Recognition	7.90 (0.45)	8.00 (0.00)	8.00 (0.00)	7.90 (0.45)	8.00 (0.00)	8.00 (0.00)	8.00 (0.00)	7.44 (1.91)	6.81 (2.20)
Oral Spelling	6.70 (2.36)	7.52 (0.77)	7.67 (0.69)	5.40 (1.14)	7.14 (0.95)	7.36 (1.13)	5.88 (1.17)	5.72 (1.56)	4.91 (1.72)
Word–Picture Matching	9.90 (0.45)	10.00 (0.00)	9.94 (0.23)	9.70 (0.73)	10.00 (0.00)	10.00 (0.00)	9.47 (1.01)	9.05 (2.44)	8.64 (2.17)
Sentences–Paragraphs	8.80 (1.00)	9.00 (1.00)	9.33 (1.28)	7.40 (1.46)	8.78 (1.05)	8.86 (1.04)	7.18 (1.13)	7.11 (2.05)	6.68 (2.08)

(Continued)

TABLE 2.2. (Continued)

	Years of education								
	0–5			6–12			13 or more		
	Age								
Subtests	16–30	31–50	51–65	16–30	31–50	51–65	16–30	31–50	51–65
Writing									
Mechanics	2.82	2.78	2.68	3.00	3.00	2.95	3.00	3.00	3.00
	(0.53)	(0.55)	(0.78)	(0.00)	(0.00)	(0.22)	(0.00)	(0.00)	(0.00)
Serial Writing	43.29	44.11	35.77	46.91	45.71	45.25	47.00	46.92	46.50
	(6.79)	(5.41)	(15.03)	(0.48)	(0.73)	(6.00)	(0.00)	(0.40)	(0.89)
Primer-Level Dictation	13.88	14.50	12.50	15.00	15.00	14.00	15.00	15.00	14.90
	(2.18)	(1.42)	(5.23)	(0.00)	(0.00)	(1.86)	(0.00)	(0.00)	(0.31)
Written Confrontation	9.82	9.78	7.54	10.00	10.00	9.10	9.94	10.00	9.20
	(0.53)	(0.94)	(3.38)	(0.00)	(0.00)	(1.02)	(0.23)	(0.00)	(1.00)
Spelling to Dictation	9.59	10.00	7.04	10.00	10.00	7.70	9.94	10.00	9.40
	(1.28)	(0.00)	(3.80)	(0.00)	(0.00)	(3.61)	(0.24)	(0.00)	(2.23)
Sentences to Dictation	10.47	10.61	9.54	12.00	12.00	11.00	12.00	12.00	11.30
	(2.45)	(2.91)	(4.23)	(0.00)	(0.00)	(1.20)	(0.00)	(0.00)	(0.40)
Narrative Writing	2.53	2.28	2.45	3.68	3.50	3.50	4.00	4.00	3.90
	(1.23)	(1.18)	(1.37)	(0.65)	(0.85)	(0.83)	(0.00)	(0.00)	(0.31)

Comments

Our results are in agreement with those obtained by Borod, Goodglass, and Kaplan (1980) in that we found BDAE sensitive to age and educational level. Although, Borod and associates also found that the educational level variable is markedly more important than the age variable, our results show markedly larger differences between educational groups. It is worth noting that the number of subjects in each educational-level group (60 subjects) was considerably larger than that used by Borod et al. (11 subjects). Also, the number of years of education for the group with the least amount of formal education was from 0 to 5 years in our study as compared with 0 to 8 years in the Borod study. The average educational level was, therefore, lower in our study.

Observe that standard deviations for the lowest educational group are higher than for the other groups. Very likely, the ceilings of the subtests were too low for higher educational groups, and hence, dispersions were minimal.

In our study, as in the study by Borod et al., age was critical in fewer subtests than was educational level. However, significant age and educational attainment differences in subtests were found that had heretofore not been reported (e.g., Body-Part Identification, Comprehension of Oral Spelling, and Spelling to Dictation). In contrast, differences were not found in subtests for which they have been reported by Borod et al. (e.g., Commands and Automatized Sequences). In most subtests, however, the results did coincide. We hypothesize that the differences on spelling tasks reflect differences between the English and Spanish writing systems. In Spanish, as a consequence of using a much more phonological writing system, spelling is heavily based on the spoken language; underlying language-cognitive processes might be different and therefore such processes are probably much more linguistically biased in Spanish than in English.

Taking into account the critical importance of the educational level, it is proposed that the various BDAE subtests have individual cutoffs according to the educational level and age of the subject. These cutoff scores are determined by each group's mean score minus two standard deviations, as presented in Table 2.3. Without using this corrected cutoff score, the likelihood of a subject being incorrectly diagnosed as aphasic might increase significantly. This would be particularly true for individuals with low educational attainment.

TABLE 2.3. Cutoff Scores According to Age and Educational Attainment for Subtests of the Boston Diagnostic Aphasia Examination

	Years of education								
	0–5			6–12			13 or more		
	Age								
Subtests	16–30	31–50	51–65	16–30	31–50	51–65	16–30	31–50	51–65
Fluency									
Phrase Length	5.0	5.0	5.0	7.0	7.0	7.0	7.0	7.0	7.0
Auditory comprehension									
Word Discrimination	55.5	54.5	46.0	72.0	69.5	57.0	72.0	72.0	72.0
Body-Part Identification	16.0	15.0	13.0	18.0	17.0	16.0	20.0	20.0	20.0
Commands	15.0	15.0	15.0	15.0	15.0	15.0	15.0	15.0	15.0
Complex Material	5.5	5.5	5.0	8.0	8.0	7.5	9.0	9.0	9.0
Naming									
Responsive Naming	27.0	25.0	23.0	29.0	29.0	29.0	30.0	30.0	30.0
Confrontation	93.0	90.0	86.0	105.0	102.0	95.0	105.0	105.0	105.0
Animal Naming	10.0	9.0	7.0	12.0	11.0	10.0	14.0	13.0	12.0
Body-Part Naming	20.0	19.0	17.0	25.5	25.5	25.0	30.0	30.0	30.0
Oral reading									
Word Reading	20.0	15.0	10.0	29.0	29.0	29.0	30.0	30.0	30.0
Oral Sentence	10.0	7.0	5.0	10.0	10.0	9.0	10.0	10.0	10.0

Repetition									
Words	10.0	10.0	10.0	10.0	10.0	10.0	10.0	10.0	10.0
High-Probability	8.0	6.5	5.0	8.0	8.0	7.0	8.0	8.0	8.0
Low-Probability	6.0	5.5	4.0	8.0	7.0	6.0	8.0	8.0	7.0
Automatic Speech									
Automatized Sequences	7.0	7.0	5.5	7.5	7.5	7.5	8.0	8.0	8.0
Reciting	2.0	2.0	2.0	2.0	2.0	2.0	2.0	2.0	2.0
Reading Comprehension									
Symbol Discrimination	8.0	7.0	5.0	10.0	9.0	8.0	10.0	10.0	9.5
Word Recognition	6.0	5.0	4.0	7.0	7.0	6.5	8.0	8.0	7.5
Oral Spelling	3.5	2.5	1.5	5.0	5.0	3.0	6.5	6.0	5.5
Word–Picture Matching	7.0	5.0	4.0	10.0	9.0	8.0	10.0	9.5	9.0
Sentences–Paragraphs	5.0	4.0	3.0	6.5	5.5	5.0	7.5	7.0	6.5
Writing									
Mechanics	2.0	1.5	1.0	3.0	2.5	2.5	3.0	3.0	3.0
Serial Writing	25.0	20.0	15.0	45.0	42.0	30.0	47.0	46.0	45.0
Primer-Level Dictation	9.5	7.5	6.0	13.0	12.0	11.0	15.0	15.0	14.0
Written Confrontation	7.0	6.0	4.0	10.0	10.0	8.0	10.0	10.0	8.0
Spelling to Dictation	6.0	4.0	2.0	9.0	8.0	7.0	10.0	10.0	9.0
Sentences to Dictation	7.0	5.0	3.0	12.0	11.0	9.0	12.0	12.0	11.0
Narrative Writing	1.5	1.0	0.5	2.5	2.5	2.0	4.0	4.0	3.0

SPANISH NAMING TEST

Background

One of the most fundamental functions of language is naming. Naming is often affected in brain damage, and indeed, virtually all aphasics present at least some naming deficits. A specific type of aphasia characterized by naming difficulties while sparing other languages functions is easily distinguished and has been named anomic or amnesic aphasia (Benson, 1979; Luria, 1966). Anomic patients present a selective difficulty among categories of words: nouns are the most severely impaired category whereas the ability to name letters and numbers is often preserved (Goodglass, Klein, Carey, & Jones, 1966).

Naming has also been observed to be a language function that is especially sensitive to the effects of aging (Bayles, 1982). Although vocabulary tends to increase well into the sixth decade of life, mild naming difficulties can be observed during the seventh decade of life (Albert, 1988). Naming disorders are always found in cases of dementia, especially in the dementia of Alzheimer's disease (Bayles, 1982). Mildly to moderately impaired Alzheimer's disease patients usually display difficulty producing the names of common objects. In the early stages of disease, patients can recognize the object, describe the function, and produce circumlocutions (Albert & Moss, 1984). With advancing disease, naming difficulties become more severe. Mild naming disorders are also readily observed in other dementia syndromes (Cummings & Benson, 1983). Furthermore, naming has been found to be one of the tasks best correlated with severity of dementia (Skelton & Jones, 1984).

Although all of the language battery tests include naming subtests, some special naming tests have been proposed. In 1978 Kaplan, Goodglass, and Weintraub published a naming test that included 60 figures with different levels of difficulty, from very easy to very complex. This test, known as the Boston Naming Test, has become particularly popular in clinical neuropsychology in North America. Items were selected in such a way that naming is unambiguous and there are no alternative names. If the subject is unable to name a particular item, a description of the item is presented; if the subject still cannot name it, a phonological cue is presented. The maximum score is 60, and norms are available for children, normal adults, the elderly, and aphasics (Borod, Goodglass, & Kaplan, 1980; Goodglass &

Kaplan, 1983; Kindlon & Garrison, 1984; LaBarge, Edwards, & Knese-vich, 1986; Van-Gorp, Satz, Kiersch, & Henry, 1986).

High reliability in this test has been reported by Huff, Collins, Corkin, and Rosen (1986). Initially, norms for the Boston Naming Test were provided in 1980 by Borod, Goodglass, and Kaplan, but norms for elderly subjects have appeared only recently. LaBarge, Edwards, and Knesevich (1986) administered the Boston Naming Test to a sample of 58 elderly normal subjects ranging from 60 to 85 years old, and Van-Gorp, Satz, Kiersch, and Henry (1986) obtained normative data for 78 normal elderly between 59 and 80 years old. Both norma-tive studies indicate that naming ability declines only slightly with age and remains fairly stable until individuals are in their seventies.

In 1986 the Boston Naming Test was translated into Spanish. In the adaptation to Spanish, some of the items were changed, but the same scoring system was maintained. However, the norms presented in the Spanish version are the norms published originally by Good-glass and Kaplan for the English version (1983) and socioeducational effects were not considered. Owing to a certain lexical diversity in Spanish among the Spanish-speaking world, some of the items are ambiguous and several different names are applicable to one object, making the test partially confusing. Some of the items are frankly unusual for a person living in Latin America. It is widely known that naming has a strong socioeducational effect (e.g., Ardila & Rosselli, 1988).

Test Description

A shortened Spanish Naming Test was developed (see Appendix A3). It consists of 15 drawn items of different levels of difficulty. Ambiguity in naming is controlled as much as possible, taking into account the lexical variations among Spanish speakers. Six of the items of the Boston Naming Test were adapted for the Spanish version, but the rest of the items were redesigned. Items such as objects, animals, cloths, and instruments are included. Semantic and phonological cueing of subjects are used when necessary. The scoring system from the Boston Naming Test was slightly modified: a score of 3 points is given when the item is correctly named, 2 points when semantic cueing is required for correct naming, 1 point when phonologic cueing is required (phonological cues are underlined in the text, Appendix A3), and 0 if correct naming is impossible even with semantic and phonologic cueing. The maximum score is 45.

Normative Data

The Spanish Naming Test was given to a sample of 346 normal subjects 55 years of age or older. Subjects were grouped according to age (56–60, 61–65, 66–70, 71–75, and over 75 years), educational level (0–5, 6–12, and more than 12 years of formal education), and sex, with 11 or 12 subjects in each cell. Table 2.4 presents the normative results. Scores were negatively correlated with age, with a decrease particularly in the low and middle educational groups.

Standard scores (percentages, percentiles, and T scores) for the following four age and educational groups are found in Appendix B, Table B3: age 55–65, with 0–5 years of formal schooling; 55–65, with more than 5 years of formal education; age 66 and over, with 0–5 years of formal education; ages 66 and over, with more than 5 years of formal education. Subjects were divided after observing that the major score differences were found between these age groups and educational level ranges.

Results in Aged and Abnormal Populations

Table 2.5 presents a general classification of naming disorders found in cases of focal brain damage and associated aphasic (or agnosic) disorder.

TABLE 2.4.   Means for the Spanish Naming Test According to Age and Education

	Age (in years)				
Education	56–60	61–65	66–70	71–75	>75
0–5 years					
Men	43.65	42.09	42.50	41.33	38.30
Women	39.88	40.10	41.00	38.50	37.10
6–12 years					
Men	44.58	43.50	42.23	42.45	39.82
Women	41.92	43.58	42.55	40.82	39.33
>12 years					
Men	44.17	44.80	44.25	44.10	43.80
Women	43.92	44.18	43.57	42.60	42.82

Note. For each correctly named test figure, 3 points were given; 2 points were given when semantic cueing was required and 1 point when phonologic cueing was required. Maximum score = 45. N = 346.

TABLE 2.5. Classification of Naming Disorders
(According to Benson and Ardila, in press)

Type of anomia	Associated aphasic (or agnosic) disorder
Word-production anomia	
Frontal anomia	Extrasylvian motor I
Articulatory initiation	Extrasylvian motor II
Articulatory reduction	Broca's aphasia
Paraphasic anomia	Conduction aphasia
Phonemic disintegration	Wernicke's aphasia
Word-selection anomia	
Semantic anomia	Extrasylvian sensory I
Special types of anomia	Extrasylvian sensory II
Category-specific anomia	
Color anomia	Color agnosia
Finger (body) anomia	Autotopagnosia
Other types	
Modality-specific anomia	
Visual anomia	Visual agnosia
Tactile anomia	Astereognosia
Auditory anomia	Auditory nonverbal agnosia
Gustatory anomia (?)	Gustatory agnosia
Olfactory anomia (?)	Olfactory agnosia
Callosal disconnection anomia	

In normal populations it is expected that the amount of naming errors will be minimal. However, naming ability is strongly correlated with educational level and tends to decrease during the seventh decade of life. Albert, Heller, and Milberg (1988) administered the Boston Naming Test to 80 healthy subjects, ranging in age from 30 to 80. Results indicated that naming ability remains stable across most of adult life, but a significant decline was observed in subjects in their seventies. Semantic and perceptual errors increased with age while lexical errors did not. A semantic deficit in Huntington's disease was demonstrated by Smith and associates (1988), using the Boston Naming Test. Knesevich, LaBarge, and Edwards (1986) used the Boston Naming Test as a predictive test of cognitive decline in Alzheimer's disease. The authors found that anomia correlated with a more rapidly progressive course of the illness. No deficits on the Boston Naming Test were found in patients with bilateral prefrontal leukotomy (Stuss & Benson, 1986).

Different types of errors have been described in testing aphasic patients. For example, in a study by Kohn and Goodglass (1985) negated responses were associated with Broca's aphasia, whole–part errors were found in frontal anomia, poor phonemic cueing was associated with Wernicke's aphasia, and anomic aphasics produced the fewest phonemic errors and the most multiword circumlocutions. In patients with Alzheimer's disease, errors are usually semantic-field errors (Martin & Fedio, 1983). The Boston Naming Test has also been frequently used to assess the recovery of naming in aphasia (e.g., Knopman, Selnes, Niccum, & Rubens, 1984).

READING AND WRITING ABILITY TESTS
FOR SPANISH SPEAKERS

Background

Different types of reading and writing disturbances after brain damage have been reported in the literature (Benson, 1985; Benson & Cummings, 1985). Traditionally, two main types of alexia are observed: literal or parietotemporal alexia, or alexia with agraphia; and verbal or occipital alexia, or alexia without agraphia (Dejerine, 1892). Benson (1977) proposed a third type of alexia, which correlates with Broca's aphasia and has been named frontal alexia. Furthermore, spatial disturbances in cases of right-hemisphere damage can disturb reading ability so severely that this deserves to be considered a fourth type of alexia, or spatial alexia (Ardila, Rosselli, & Pinzon, 1989; Benson & Ardila, in press). Table 2.6 presents a general classification

TABLE 2.6.   Classification of Alexias

Central alexia (parietotemporal alexia)
Posterior alexia (occipital alexia)
Anterior alexia (frontal alexia)
Spatial alexia (right-hemisphere alexia)
Other varieties of alexias (associated with other lesion locations):
Aphasic alexias
Hemialexia
Phonological alexia
Surface alexia
Deep alexia

of alexias. Table 2.7 presents the main characteristics and associated clinical findings for the four basic varieties of alexias.

Writing disturbances usually are divided into two main groups: those depending on a fundamental language disorder (aphasic agraphias) and those depending not on a fundamental linguistic disorder (nonaphasic agraphias) but on motor disturbances, spatial impairments, or other associated disorders. Table 2.8 presents a general classification of agraphias.

Reading and writing disorders are not completely equivalent across different languages. Difficulties in reading and writing depend to a great extent on the specific writing system. Japanese is the best example of dissociation (Sasanuma & Fujimura, 1971), but many other examples can be found. For instance, Luria (1964) describes a bilingual (Russian and French) patient with a dissociation for reading French and Russian. Recently, great interest has been accorded the so-called "psycholinguistic" models of reading disturbances, especially those developed for English (Marshall & Newcombe, 1973; Roeltgen, 1985). However, the applicability of these models to other languages, like Spanish, has been challenged (Ardila, Rosselli & Pinzon, 1989; Ardila, 1991). It has been argued that the cognitive processes underlying reading (and writing) in English and in Spanish are not equivalent.

Testing Reading and Writing

Usually, reading ability is examined in conjunction with oral language testing. Some basic reading and writing tasks are routinely included in standard neuropsychological evaluations. Reading is usually tested simultaneously with writing. Table 2.9 presents a summary of the main tasks used in reading and writing assessment.

The reading and writing of letters, syllables, words, logotomes, and sentences correspond to progressively more complex levels of functioning. Different types of letters (uppercase, lowercase, cursive) should be included in this assessment. It is important to use words with different levels of difficulty. The reading of highly meaningful words (such as the name of the patient and the name of his or her country) is frequently preserved in alexic patients. Matching words with different types of writing is important in the evaluation of alexia, since this task is virtually impossible to perform for those with central alexia.

Reading comprehension is tested by having the subject match words and objects and follow written commands. More complex

TABLE 2.7. Differential Features of the Four Alexias

Area of functioning	Parietotemporal	Occiptal	Frontal	Spatial
Main characteristics				
1. Reading	Total alexia	Primarily verbal	Primarily literal	Spatial alexia
2. Writing	Severe agraphia except copying	Mild or no agraphia	Severe agraphia, including copying	Spatial agraphia
3. Copying	Slavish	Slavish	Poor, clumsy, omissions	Left hemineglect
4. Letter-naming	Anomia for letters	Normal	Anomia for letters	Normal
5. Comprehension of spelled words	Failed	Good	Poor	Good
6. Spelling out loud	Failed	Good	Poor	Good
Associated findings				
1. Language	Fluent aphasia	Normal or mild anomia	Nonfluent aphasia	Normal
2. Motor	Mild paresis	Normal	Hemiplegia	Left hemiparesis
3. Sensory	Often hemisensory loss	Normal	Usually mild sensory loss	Usually hemisensory loss
4. Visual field	May or may not have visual field defects	Right hemianopsia	Normal	Usually left hemianopsia
5. Gerstmann's syndrome	Frequent	Absent	Absent	Absent

Note. Adapted from "Alexia," by D. F. Benson in J. A. M. Frederiks (ed.), Handbook of Clinical Neurology: Vol. 45. Clinical Neuropsychology (pp. 433–435), 1985, Amsterdam: Elsevier.

TABLE 2.8.   Classification of Agraphias

Aphasic agraphias	Nonaphasic agraphias
Agraphia in Broca's aphasia	Motor agraphias
Agraphia in Wernicke's aphasia	Paretic agraphia
Agraphia in conduction aphasia	Hypokinetic agraphia
Agraphia in other aphasias	Hyperkinetic agraphia
Phonological agraphia	Pure agraphia
Lexical agraphia	Apraxic agraphia
Deep agraphia	Spatial agraphia

levels of functioning are required in the silent reading of paragraphs after which subjects are asked to report what they have read or to answer specific questions about the material.

Spelling aloud and recognizing spelled words are tasks that can be very difficult for people with specific brain pathology, since this deficit is correlated with specific types of alexias. In bilingual (and polyglot) subjects, reading should be tested for both (or all of the) languages because reading abilities for the different languages may differ.

Spontaneous writing is usually tested by asking the subject to write a report about a particular topic (e.g., weather, work) or by presenting the subject with a figure to describe. Subtle writing disturbances can then be observed.

Testing reading and writing with other symbolic systems is not frequently used. However, when possible, this approach may yield

TABLE 2.9.   Main Tasks in Reading
and Writing Assessment

Reading and writing	Spelling
Letters	Comprehension of oral spelling
Syllables	Spelling of words
Logotomes	Arranging the letters of a word
Words	Matching different types of writing
Sentences	Reading comprehension
Paragraphs	Matching words with objects
Automatic writing	Commands
Signature	Paragraph comprehension
Days of the week	Spontaneous writing
Ideographic reading	

particularly interesting results and includes the reading and writing of musical notes and chemical symbols and recognizing logotypes.

Test Description

Tests for reading and writing for Spanish speakers were designed (see Appendix A4 and A5) and include the following tasks:

1. Reading Ability Test
   Reading of letters
   Reading of syllables
   Reading of logotomes
   Reading of words
   Reading of sentences
   Comprehension of written commands
   Text reading
   Text comprehension
2. Writing Ability Test
   Writing of letters
   Writing of syllables
   Writing of words
   Writing of sentences
   Change from cursive to printing
   Change from printing to cursive
   Change from uppercase to lowercase letters
   Change from lowercase to uppercase
   Written description of a picture

Normative Data

The reading and writing abilities tests were given to 180 neurologically normal adults, divided into three educational groups (0–5, 6–12, and more than 12 years of formal education) and three age ranges (16–30, 31–50, and 51–65 years). Statistically significant differences were found only for educational level ($F = 35.60$; $df = 2$; $p<.001$) in the Reading Ability Test for Spanish Speakers. Interaction between age and education level was significant ($F = 2.52$; $df = 4$; $p<.05$). Table 2.10 presents the average number of errors in each group; a score correcting for a subject's educational level is proposed.

In the Writing Ability Test for Spanish Speakers, statistically significant differences according to educational level were found ($F =$

TABLE 2.10. Average Total Number of Errors
by Normal Subjects in the Reading Ability
Test for Spanish Speakers According
to Age and Educational Level (N = 180)

	Age (years)			
Education	16–30	31–50	51–65	Average
0–5 years	7.40	4.00	4.45	5.28
6–12 years	3.80	2.30	2.55	2.88
>12 years	1.00	0.60	0.70	0.76
Average	4.07	2.30	2.57	2.97

Note. The following scores are proposed to correct for a
subject's educational level:

Years of education	Correction score
<6 years	−6
6–12 years	−3
>12 years	0

13.95; $df = 2$; $p<.0001$). The interaction between age and education
was also significant ($F = 4.06$; $df = 4$; $p<.01$). Table 2.11 presents the
average number of errors in the different groups; a correction score is
proposed. Results of these tests in brain-damaged individuals are
presented elsewhere (see Ardila, Rosselli & Pinzon, 1989).

SPANISH REPETITION TEST

Background

Verbal repetition represents a basic linguistic ability, and virtually all language tests include a section of repetition (e.g., Goodglass & Kaplan, 1972; Kertesz, 1979). Furthermore, it is believed that
some aphasic disturbances can be distinguished solely on the basis of
the patient's ability to repeat. The ability to repeat is preserved in the
"transylvian" (or transcortical) aphasias whereas it is impaired in the
"conduction," or afferent motor, aphasias (Benson & Ardila, in press;
Benson, 1979; Kertesz, 1979, 1985; Luria, 1966, 1976a).

Normative Data

A repetition test for Spanish speakers (Appendix A6), which
contains the following sections, was developed:

TABLE 2.11. Average Total Number of Errors
by Normal Subjects in the Writing Ability
Test for Spanish Speakers According
to Age and Educational Level ($N = 180$)

	Age (years)			
Education	16–30	31–50	51–65	Average
0–5 years	5.55	2.10	2.05	3.23
6–12 years	1.00	1.30	1.25	1.18
>12 years	0.30	0.45	0.30	0.35
Average	2.28	1.28	1.20	1.59

Note. The following scores are proposed to correct for a
subject's educational level:

Years of education	Correction score
<6 years	−3
6–12 years	−1
>12 years	0

1. Phoneme repetition
2. Syllable repetition
3. Repetition of logotomes
4. Repetition of minimal pairs
5. Repetition of words
6. Repetition of phrases and sentences

The test was given to 180 neurologically intact subjects, matched according to three variables: educational level, age, and sex. The scoring system was based on the total number of errors on all six parts of the test. Table 2.12 presents the results for this population.

A three-way analysis of variance disclosed that educational level had a significant effect on results ($F = 39.94$; $df = 2$; $p<.001$), but no age ($F = 0.967$; $df = 2$; $p = NS$) or sex ($F = 1.76$; $df = 1$; $p = NS$) effects were observed. Further, no interactions were significant. The average number of errors were 3.68 for the highest educational level and 12.48 for the lowest. A correction score is proposed according to the subject's educational level.

A special analysis was done with regard to the maximum number of words in a sentence an individual could repeat. Table 2.13 presents the average results. An educational level, but not age, effect is observed. On average, a neurologically normal person can repeat a sentence of 15 ± 3 words.

TABLE 2.12. Average Total Number
of Errors by Normal Subjects on the Spanish
Repetition Test According to Age and
Educational Level ($N = 180$)

	Age (years)			
Education	16–30	31–50	51–65	Average
0–5 years	14.85	13.40	9.20	12.48
6–12 years	9.10	6.60	10.70	8.80
>12 years	3.30	3.75	4.00	3.68
Average	9.08	7.92	7.99	8.82

Note. The following scores are proposed to correct for a
subject's educational level:

Years of education	Correction score
<6 years	−13
6–12 years	−9
>12 years	−4

Results for Brain-Damaged Populations

Deficits in repetition have been associated with conduction
aphasia or afferent motor aphasia. Conduction aphasia, first described by Wernicke in 1874, is characterized by fluent paraphasic
(usually literal) conversational speech, near-normal comprehension,
and repetition disturbance of a significant degree; it often includes
(1) naming disturbances (from literal paraphasic contamination to
total inability to produce the appropriate word); (2) reading disturbances (comprehension is better than reading aloud); (3) writing dis-

TABLE 2.13. Average Maximum Number
of Words Repeated in a Sentence by Normal
Subjects on the Spanish Repetition Test
According to Age and Educational Level

	Age (years)		
Education	16–30	31–50	51–65
0–5 years	12	13	13
6–12 years	14	14	14
>12 years	17	17	17

turbances (from mild spelling difficulties to profound agraphia); (4) ideomotor apraxia (buccofacial and limb); and (5) elementary neurological abnormalities, namely, some right hemiparesis and cortical sensory loss (Benson, Sheretana, Bouchard, Segarra, Price, & Geschwind, 1973). Furthermore, phonological approximations to the word sought and self-corrections are often observed in the patient's speech.

The principal defect in conduction aphasia is that of repetition. However, different mechanisms may underlie the defect of repetition. These would depend on the level of language alteration during the repetition, for example, whether short or long elements are repeated, whether automatic elements or meaningless sequences are used, whether nominative or grammatical elements are included, and so forth. These considerations have led to the proposition that there are at least two different kinds of conduction aphasia: efferent and afferent (Kertesz, 1979, 1985), and reproduction and repetition (Caplan, Vanier, & Baker, 1986; Shallice & Warrington, 1977). The first type, considered to be the result of disorganization in the phonemic content of words, can be seen in the repetition of words or short elements. This is of parietal origin. The second type is a consequence of alterations in verbal memory; it involves the repetition of long sequences and is of temporal origin.

Caramazza, Basili, Koller, and Berndt (1981) reported that the conduction aphasia syndrome should be divided into two subgroups on the basis of the patient's ability to choose and produce phonemes in his or her expressive language. When there is a deficit in repetition without significant speech-output problems, the defect is in auditory verbal short-term memory. Benson and associates (1973) also distinguished two kinds of conduction aphasia: suprasylvian (parietal) and subsylvian (temporal), the first of which is associated with ideomotor apraxia. Luria (1966, 1970, 1976a) noted that what has classically been called conduction aphasia corresponds to two different language defects. He used the term *afferent motor aphasia* for the parietal type of conduction aphasia and considered this aphasia to be an alteration in the structure of word sounds in their articulatory unit (articuleme) with an underlying apraxic defect. The second kind of conduction aphasia (temporal) is included within acoustic–amnesic aphasia and depends on a verbal memory defect.

It would therefore seem reasonably well established that two different mechanisms can lead to defects in language repetition. Moreover, defects in language repetition are reflected in different ways. In cases of parietal (and insular) conduction aphasia, defects become apparent in the repetition of even short linguistic segments and are particularly evident in the repetition of logotomes. In the temporal type of conduction aphasia, deficits become evident in the repetition of long segments. In the first case, repetition deficits are associated with apraxia while in the second case repetition impairments are associated with verbal memory defects. However, the defect in repetition in the case of parietal conduction aphasia has been interpreted in different ways, namely, in terms of disconnection (Damasio & Damasio, 1980, 1983; Geschwind, 1975) or in terms of an apraxic defect (Brown, 1975; Luria, 1970, 1976a; Vinarskaya, 1971). Given the latter interpretation, conduction aphasia has been called an "ideomotor apraxia of speech" (Brown, 1975) or a "kinesthetic apraxia of speech" (Luria, 1976a). It seems reasonable to suppose that the language repetition deficits in parietal conduction aphasia and in ideomotor apraxia might be based on the same basic disturbances (Ardila & Rosselli, 1989).

SPANISH PHONEMIC DISCRIMINATION TEST

Background

Phonological discrimination represents a fundamental ability in language recognition. Disorders in phonemic discrimination have been named word deafness (Gazzaniga, Glass, Sarno & Posner, 1973), verbal auditory agnosia (Bauer & Rubens, 1985), auditory receptive aphasia (Walsh, 1987), or acoustic agnostic aphasia (Luria, 1966, 1973). Phonemic discrimination deficits can be found mainly in fluent aphasics and are correlated with language comprehension difficulties.

Testing for phonemic discrimination is routine in aphasia assessment. A phonemic discrimination test must be given in the patient's native language. Although some phonemes are found across different languages, the phonemic repertoire in different languages varies. In Spanish there are 23 phonemes, in English about 40. Table 2.14 presents the phonological organization of the Spanish language.

Avila (1976) developed a Spanish phonemic discrimination test for the diagnosis of aphasics, taking into account the phonological particularities of the Spanish spoken in Latin America. Ardila, Montanes, Caro, Delgado, and Buckingham (1989) analyzed the phonological transformations found in Spanish-speaking aphasics.

TABLE 2.14. The Spanish Phonological System

	Labials		Dentals		Alveolars		Palatals		Velars	
	vl	vd	vl	vd	vl	vd	vl	vd	vl	vd
Stops	p	b	t	d					k	g
Affricates							tʃ			
Nasals	m				n		ɲ			
Flap							ŕ			
Trill							ŕ			
Fricatives	f				s				x	
Laterals						l		ĺ		

Note: There are 17 consonantal phonemes (the voiced, lateral, palatal /ĺ/ is found in some scattered regions, but in general, this phoneme is fading from the language. The phoneme /x/ (voiced, velar, fricative) is lowering articulatorily into the glottal region. The voiced oral stop phonemes /b/, /d/, and /g/ have very weakly articulated fricative allophones in intervocalic position. There are five simple vowel phonemes at cardinal points: /a/, /e/, /i/, /u/, and /o/. The letters y and w function as semiconsonants when they are the nontonic left member of diphthongs, such as the words "tyene" and "kwanto", while they function as semivowels when they are the nontonic right member of diphthongs such as [peyne] and [kawsa]. They function as full consonants when they occur alone with no contiguous consonant.

Test Description

A test for phonemic discrimination can include a sample of minimal pairs (minimal phonological difference conveying meaning). Table 2.15 presents a sample of minimal pairs for Spanish. Meaningless syllables and/or meaningful words can be used. However, it is more convenient to use meaningful words since the instructions are easier for the examiner to present and easier for the patient to understand.

A test for Spanish phonemic discrimination, based on Avila

TABLE 2.15. Some Examples
of Minimal Pairs in Spanish

Word pairs	Phonemes	Opposition involved
Pala–Bala, Peso–Beso	/p/-/b/	Unvoiced–Voiced
Higo–Hijo, Garra–Jarra	/g/-/x/	Stop–Fricative
Toro–Coro, Tuna–Cuna	/k/-/t/	Dental–Velar
Fuente–Puente, Farra–Parra	/p/-/f/	Stop–Fricative
Caro–Carro, Moro–Morro	/r/-/r/	Flap–Trill
Pata–Mata, Capa–Cama	/p/-/m/	Stop–Nasal
Dia–Tia, Viendo–Viento	/d/-/t/	Unvoiced–Voiced

(1976), was constructed. The test is composed of 40 word pairs corresponding to phonological minimal pairs in Spanish (see Appendix A7). The subject is instructed to indicate if the two words are the same or different; there are 20 same and 20 different word pairs. The examiner reads the pair of words, and the subject has to respond "same" or "different" (or "yes" or "no" or to move the head in correspondence). Pronunciation must be clear (or a tape can be used). The subject should not see the examiner's mouth movements during the reading of the words (the examiner can stand behind the subject, or subjects can be instructed to close their eyes). The subject's response for each word pair is registered, and the percentage of correct responses is determined.

Normative Data

A normal person is expected to present a nearly perfect performance in a phonemic discrimination task, particularly when meaningful words are used. Benton, Hamsher, Varney, and Spreen (1983) reported that 90% of normal people achieved a success rate of more than 83% in a phonemic discrimination task for nonsense syllables. Rosselli, Ardila, and Rosas (1990) found that phoneme discrimination of meaningful words was strongly influenced by educational level. Literate people present a virtually perfect performance up to the seventh decade of life, when about 2% of errors are expected. This percentage tends to increase in higher age ranges.

Observed errors during aging are influenced by two factors: hypoacusis and memory deficits. When performing the phonemic discrimination task, elderly subjects forget the first syllable or word when the second one is presented. Memory deficits and, particularly, hypoacusis, can be partially responsible for the lower scores observed in the elderly. However, it may be reasonable to assume that phonemic discrimination itself is also affected by age.

Illiteracy is associated with low performance in virtually every language task, including phonemic discrimination, where errors were observed in every age range studied. However, the percentage of errors was found to be approximately the same up to the sixth decade of life, after which time errors increased in illiterates. Some additional factors may contribute to the low performance in neuropsychological tasks in illiterates, including lack of familiarity with testing situations, underestimation of the importance of "artificial" and nonsense tasks (and, consequently, the production of rather random answers), aversion to being tested and measured, and embarrassment with testing situations.

Results in Brain-Damaged Patients

Difficulties in phonemic discrimination, particularly word deafness, have been associated with Wernicke's aphasia. Benton and associates (1983) observed that 80% of their aphasic patients presented deficits in phonemic discrimination (in about half of them performance was near chance level). Phonemic discrimination deficits are highly correlated with language comprehension deficits. Phonemic discrimination defects are usually found in cases of left temporal damage (Luria, 1966). Various studies have emphasized that language comprehension deficits are at least partially due to phonemic discrimination failures (e.g., Basso, Casati, & Vignolo, 1977; Blumstein, Baker, & Goodglass, 1977; Miceli, Gainotti, Caltagirone & Masullo, 1980; Varney & Benton, 1979). Phonemic discrimination is considered to be a necessary but not sufficient basis for intact oral verbal comprehension in aphasic patients (Benton et al., 1983).

Luria (1970) found the phonemic imperception of acoustic-agnostic aphasia followed damage to the superior temporal lobe. Others also noted that unilateral lesions causing pure word deafness consistently involve Heschl's gyri and/or surrounding areas (Gazzaniga et al., 1973; Benson, 1979). Liepmann and Storck's (1902) case of word deafness had a left temporal subcortical lesion that included the posterior insula. Kertesz (1983) reported a case of word deafness with damage in the superior temporal gyrus and middle portions of the temporal operculum involving the posterior insula.

SPANISH GRAMMAR TEST

Background

Morphology is the study of patterns of word formation (inflections, derivations, and compositions) and refers to the construction of words in a language. Syntax refers to the rules applied to the construction of phrases and sentences. The sequence of words in a sentence depends on the particular language and on the specific communication intention. Different languages employ different word orders, although some word orders are more frequently found across different languages. Languages vary with regard to the rigidity of the word order: English is considered a language with a strict word order while Spanish is considered to have a very flexible word order. Grammar represents the rules that govern the structure of language; therefore, grammar includes morphology and syntax.

Agrammatism involves the disruption of grammatical structure in language (Kean, 1985). Agrammatic aphasics have unusual difficulty using and understanding grammatical morphemes (connectors and affixes) but fewer problems in the use and understanding of lexical morphemes. The disruption of grammatical structure often appears to be telegraphic (e.g., "The man walks in the street" becomes "Man street"). Phrase length is decreased but semantic content increases, with meaning being expressed by only a few words. Verbs are incorrectly used in tense and person, while nouns are the best-preserved language element.

Paragrammatism (or dyssyntaxia) is a grammatical deviation characterized by a verbal output that violates the normative rules of the common morphosyntactic convention (Lecours, Trepagnier, Naesser, & Lavelle-Huynh, 1983). It results from (1) overuse of grammatical elements (particularly connectors) associated with a decrease in nouns, (2) erroneous selection of grammatical elements, and (3) an absence of definitive limits in the sentence, correlated with an excessive verbal output (logorrhea).

Agrammatism represents one of the most salient clinical features in aphasic language, particularly in Broca's aphasia. This observation has been repeatedly confirmed in the literature. Agrammatism has been differentiated from the paragrammatism found in Wernicke's aphasia. Nonfluent agrammatic patients show very poor comprehension of syntax. Howes (1967), who studied the relative frequency of lexical and grammatical words in different types of aphasia, found that grammatical units are less frequently found in Broca's aphasia. Grammatical units were normally found (and even sometimes found in excess) in Wernicke's aphasia. Goodglass, Quafasel, and Timberlake (1964) observed that most utterances produced by nonfluent aphasics include only one or two words, mainly nouns. Goodglass, Fodor, and Schulhoff (1967) hypothesized that omission of grammatical connectors in agrammatic patients is related to the salience and position of the grammatical particles. Goodglass and Huner (1970) compared the oral and written productions of aphasics and found that agrammatism (telegraphic style) in Broca aphasics is observed in both oral language and written production. Each subject's syntactic deviations were qualitatively similar in his or her oral and written language. Thus, the analysis of grammar in aphasic patients represents a crucial aspect of any language assessment.

Test Description

A test of grammar for Spanish-speaking aphasics was designed (see Appendix A8). The test includes the following sections:

1. Spontaneous Language (a description of Plate 1 from the Boston Diagnostic Aphasia Examination [Goodglass & Kaplan, 1972]; see Figure 2.1):
   1.1. Number of nouns
   1.2. Number of verbs
   1.3. Number of adjectives
   1.4. Number of grammatical connnectors
   1.5. Total number of words
2. Sentence Completion:Verbs (total = 19)
3. Sentence Completion:Prepositions (total = 27)

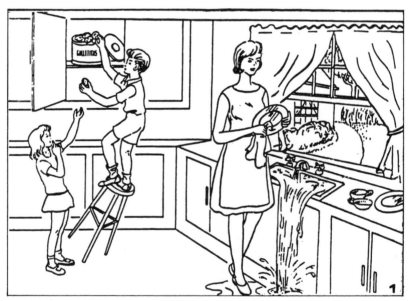

FIGURE 2.1. Plate 1 from the Boston Diagnostic Aphasia Examination. This figure was used in the Spontaneous Language section of the Spanish Grammar Test. (Reprinted by permission of Lea and Febiger, Malvern, Pennsylvania.)

4. Concordance:Use of Articles (total = 12)
5. Concordance:Use of Adjectives (total = 20)
6. Grammatical Transformations:
    6.1. Verbs to nouns (total = 4)
    6.2. Nouns and adjectives to verbs (total = 11)
    6.3. Antonyms (total = 12)
7. Comparative Constructions (total = 12)
8. Coordinate Sentences (total = 10)

The Spontaneous Language section of the test (description of Plate 1 from the Boston Diagnostic Aphasia Examination; Goodglass & Kaplan, 1972) was given to 180 neurologically normal adults divided according to age (16–30, 31–50, and 51–56 years old), educational level (0–5, 6–12, and more than 12 years of formal education), and sex.

Normative Data

In the Picture Description subtest of the Spontaneous Language section, it was observed that the number of nouns, verbs, adjectives, and grammatical connections increased across educational level (Tables 2.16–2.19). That is, language production increased as the subject's schooling level increased. Consequently, the total number of words used for describing the plate significantly increased across educational level ranges (Table 2.20). Changes observed across ages were inconsistent; most frequently, the youngest group presented the highest language production.

Some differences between sexes were significant. Men used an

TABLE 2.16.   Mean Number of Nouns
Obtained by Normal Subjects
on the Picture Description Subtest
of the Spanish Grammar Test (N = 180)

Education	Age (years)			
	16–30	31–50	51–65	Average
0–5 years	7.50	4.45	4.40	5.45
6–12 years	6.95	6.15	8.35	7.15
>12 years	9.75	8.55	6.25	8.18
Average	8.07	6.38	6.33	6.93

TABLE 2.17.   Mean Number of Verbs
Obtained by Normal Subjects
on the Picture Description Subtest
of the Spanish Grammar Test ($N = 180$)

| | Age (years) | | | |
Education	16–30	31–50	51–65	Average
0–5 years	7.30	1.95	4.00	4.42
6–12 years	9.25	3.30	6.55	6.37
>12 years	7.90	8.95	5.90	7.58
Average	8.15	4.73	5.48	6.12

TABLE 2.18.   Mean Number of Adjectives
Obtained by Normal Subjects
on the Picture Description Subtest
of the Spanish Grammar Test ($N = 180$)

| | Age (years) | | | |
Education	16–30	31–50	51–65	Average
0–5 years	1.40	2.05	0.65	1.37
6–12 years	1.60	2.45	3.50	2.52
>12 years	2.05	5.05	1.80	2.97
Average	1.68	3.18	1.98	2.28

TABLE 2.19.   Mean Number of Grammatical
Connectors Obtained by Normal Subjects
on the Picture Description Subtest
of the Spanish Grammar Test ($N = 180$)

| | Age (years) | | | |
Education	16–30	31–50	51–65	Average
0–5 years	8.85	5.50	6.15	6.83
6–12 years	11.35	8.50	7.10	8.98
>12 years	15.55	10.30	9.55	11.80
Average	11.92	8.10	7.60	9.21

TABLE 2.20.   Mean Total Number of Words
Obtained by Normal Subjects
on the Picture Description Subtest
of the Spanish Grammar Test (N = 180)

Education	Age (years)			
	16–30	31–50	51–65	Average
0–5 years	25.05	13.95	15.20	18.06
6–12 years	29.15	20.40	25.50	25.01
>12 years	35.25	32.85	23.50	30.53
Average	29.81	22.40	21.40	24.53

average of 22.84 words for describing the plate, while women employed 26.24 (p<.01). Differences with regard to the number of nouns (6.56 and 7.30, respectively, for men and women), verbs (5.70 and 6.54), and adjectives (2.12 and 2.44) were not significant. Differences in the use of grammatical connectors (8.46 and 9.66, respectively, for men and women) were statistically significant (p<.02).

Any native speaker of a language is expected to correctly handle the basic grammar. However, the amount of language used in a particular verbal task significantly varies according to educational level and age.

TOKEN TEST (ABBREVIATED VERSION)

Background

The Token Test is based on the assumption that communicative abilities can be disrupted even when the patient appears able to relate to others. The possibility exists that an aphasic individual could actually have problems in understanding or expressing symbolic logic, for example. Nevertheless, the test is relatively easy for minimally educated individuals (Boller and Vignolo, 1966).

Test Description

The Token Test, designed in 1962 by De Renzi and Vignolo has become one of the most widely used tests for language comprehension. It consists of 20 tokens that come in two shapes (circles and squares), two sizes (large and small), and five colors (red, green, yellow, blue, and white). The tokens are arranged in front of the patient, and the patient is asked to follow 62 commands, given in five sections of the test and organized by increasing level of difficulty. Initially, only single commands are included (e.g., "Touch the red circle"). Some of the commands, however, require an understanding of three semantic categories (e.g., "touch the large white square"). Double commands with two ("touch the blue square and the white circle") and three ("touch the small white square and the large red square") semantic categories, are presented later. An understanding of spatial relationships is included in the last section (e.g., "Put the blue circle under the white square").

This test has been extensively used in the assessment of aphasic patients (Lezak, 1983). Some further modifications have been introduced by others (Benton & Hamsher, 1976; Boller & Vignolo, 1966; Spellacy & Spreen, 1969; Spreen & Benton, 1969). In 1978, De Renzi and Faglioni studied the effects of age and education on Token Test scores. They developed a short version of the test using only 36 items. This version is divided into five sections. The first section includes seven items while the fifth and last section includes 17 items. Sections 2, 3, and 4 each include only four items. De Renzi and Faglioni recommend the adjustment of scores for education (for 3–6 years of education one point is added to the score, for 10–12 years one point is subtracted, for 13–16 years two points are subtracted, and for more than 17 years three points are subtracted). They propose a cutoff score of 29 points between normals and brain-damaged patients.

Normative Data

A Spanish translation of the De Renzi and Faglioni shortened version of the Token Test was prepared (see Appendix A9) and administered to 180 neurologically normal adults divided into three educational groups (0–5, 6–12, and more than 12 years of formal education) and three age ranges (16–30, 31–50, and 51–65 years old). Table 2.21 presents the average scores and the standard deviations in each group. A correction score is proposed according to the individual's age and educational level (Table 2.22).

TABLE 2.21. Means and Standard
Deviations (in parentheses) of Scores
of Normal Subjects on the Token Test
According to Age and Educational Level

Age	Education (years)		
	0–5	6–12	12+
16–30 yrs	34.66	35.11	35.95
	(1.49)	(1.40)	(0.20)
31–50 yrs	34.48	34.62	35.50
	(1.77)	(1.59)	(0.89)
51–65 yrs	34.07	34.21	35.41
	(1.93)	(1.27)	(1.32)

Results in Brain-Damaged Patients

The Token Test has been extensively used in the clinical assessment of aphasic patients. It is useful in discriminating mild aphasics and normals (Kertesz, 1986). Aphasic patients with auditory comprehension deficits have a tendency to confuse colors and shapes (Lezak, 1983), and global aphasics perform very poorly on this test (Collins, 1986). Memory deficits are commonly observed in a subject's failure to perform the required number of tasks in the instructions. The patient with short-term memory deficits may perform commands given in a short sentence but present difficulties in following long sentences. Aphasics with comprehension deficits present memory deficits also. Perseveration is frequently seen in brain-damaged patients.

TABLE 2.22. Age and Educational
Level Score Correction (Mean Minus
One Standard Deviation) for
the Token Test (Abbreviated Version)

Age	Education (years)		
	0–5	6–12	>12
16–30 yrs	3	2	0
31–50 yrs	3	3	1
51–65 yrs	4	3	2

VERBAL FLUENCY TEST

Background

Language fluency is usually measured by the number of words produced in a particular category within a certain time limit (most frequently, 1 minute). Age, sex, and educational level have been found to influence performance on tests measuring this variable (Ardila & Rosselli, 1988; Benton & Hamsher, 1976; Rosselli, Ardila, & Rosas, 1990; Wertz, 1979). Two main categories of words have been used in the assessment of fluency: semantic (words belonging to a particular category, such as animals or fruits) and phonological (words beginning with a particular phoneme).

A verbal fluency test consisting of three word-naming trials was developed as part of the Multilingual Aphasia Examination (Benton and Hamsher, 1976). Since the letters usually employed are *F*, *A*, and *S*, this test is sometimes called the FAS Test (Benton & Hamsher, 1976). Frequency ranges have been reported by the authors for several languages (English, French, German, and Spanish). The number of words generated that begin with a particular letter is expected to be 15 ± 5 in normal populations. However, this score is sensitive to age, educational level, and sex (Ardila & Rosselli, 1989), and a correction score has been proposed for these three variables.

The Stanford-Binet Intelligence Battery included a section in which the subject was asked to name as many animals as possible. This test was included as part of the Boston Diagnostic Examination (Goodglass & Kaplan, 1979, 1983). Normative data indicate that ten-year-olds name twelve different animals in one minute, the average adult about 18.

Procedure

The examiner asks the subject to name as many words as possible beginning with a particular letter or belonging to a particular semantic group (usually animals, vegetables, or fruits); one word is given as an example. In the phonological version, the subject is advised that proper names are not allowed. The examiner times the subject and writes down all the words generated, even if they are wrong. After 1 minute the test is terminated, and the examiner says, "Now let's try with the letter A; ready?"

To obtain a score, one counts the number of correct words. It is also advisable to score separately the following types of mistakes: (1) repetition (the same word is produced on more than one occasion); (2) intrusions (a word belonging to another category is offered (e.g., when naming fruits, the subject names vegetables); (3) perseveration (the patient provides words belonging to a category previously used); (4) derivative words (the subject produces a word and then begins to say other words with the same lexical root—e.g., sun, sunny); and (5) proper names. Appendix A10 presents an answer sheet that can be used.

Normative Data

Two different normative studies on verbal fluency were completed in order to analyze the influence of educational level and age on performance. A test with semantic (animals and fruits) and phonological (F, A, S) categories grouped according to age (56 and older) was initially administered to 200 normal subjects belonging to two extreme educational groups (illiterate and professional). For all subjects, phonological search was more difficult than semantic search. Illiterates had extreme difficulty in phonological search, and their performance on this section was two to three times lower than in semantic search (Table 2.23). The scores correspond to average per category.

The effect of aging on verbal fluency was analyzed using a sample of 346 normal elderly subjects. It was observed that this ability was very sensitive to the effect of normal aging. Performance by subjects in

TABLE 2.23. Average Number of Words Generated by Normal Subjects Differing on Educational Level and Age for Verbal Fluency Subtests ($N = 200$)

Education level	Age				
	56–60	61–65	66–70	71–75	>75
Illiterates					
Semantic	11.15	11.25	10.62	10.30	9.65
Phonologic	4.90	4.25	3.15	3.76	2.93
Professionals					
Semantic	17.75	18.47	18.02	18.27	16.77
Phonologic	15.33	16.66	17.15	17.15	16.11

TABLE 2.24. Mean Scores of Normal Subjects
on Verbal Fluency Test Semantic (and Phonological)
Subtest (N = 346) by Age and Education Level

Education	Age				
	56–69	61–65	66–70	71–75	>75
0–5 yrs	12.82	12.21	11.21	11.28	9.45
	(9.41)	(8.40)	(7.29)	(7.27)	(7.02)
6–12 yrs	16.00	15.93	13.39	12.70	10.95
	(12.29)	(12.10)	(9.92)	(9.34)	(7.21)
>12	16.10	16.15	15.81	13.77	11.72
	(13.36)	(12.92)	(12.54)	(12.43)	(9.08)

their late seventies was about 50% lower than for those in their late fifties. Decrease in productivity was similar for semantic and phonological categories.

Norms (percentages, percentiles, and T scores) were obtained for the following four educational and age groups and are found in Appendix B4: 55–65 years and 0–5 years of formal education; 55–65 years and more than 5 years of formal education; over 65 years and 0–5 years of formal education; and over 65 years and more than 5 years of formal education.

Results in Brain-Damaged Patients

Verbal fluency can be impaired after frontal lobe damage, particularly left-frontal damage (Benton, 1968; Crockett, Bilsker, Hurwitz, & Kozak, 1986; Hecaen & Ruel, 1981; Stuss & Benson, 1986). This group of patients is impaired in phonological categories but apparently not in semantic categories (Newcombe, 1969). Left-frontal damage patients produce, on the average, almost one-third fewer words on phonological fluency tests than patients with right frontal lesions. Patients with bilateral damage present as impaired as left-hemisphere damage patients. Frontal patients can also present with perseverations, difficulty maintaining the required category (intrusions), repetition of word errors, and the frequent use of derivative words.

In dementia, mainly of the Alzheimer's disease type, there is reduced ability to generate words (Miller & Hague, 1975; Stuss & Benson, 1986), especially according to phonological category. Rosen (1980) found that both elderly control subjects and mildly demented patients generated more words for semantic (animal) than for phonological categories. Patients in moderate or severe stages of dementia did equally poorly on both fluency tests. Demented patients usually produce less than half the words produced by elderly control subjects. In normal elderly subjects, eventually perseverative errors are observed, particularly after the age of 70.

A decrement in verbal fluency is also observed in aphasia but this depends a great deal on the type of aphasia and its severity (Lezak, 1983). According to Newcombe (1969), verbal fluency is an excellent task for discriminating right- from left-hemisphere damage.

CALCULATION ABILITY TEST

Background

Acalculia represents one of the most complex neuropsychological syndromes. Henschen (1920) first described a disturbance of calculating produced by a focal lesion of the brain. Berger (1926) distinguished between a primary and a secondary acalculia. Secondary acalculia refers to a defect in calculation ability derived from a fundamental cognitive deficit such as memory or attention. Hecaen, Angelergues and Houiller (1961) identified three different types of calculation disorder: (1) alexia and agraphia for numbers, (2) spatial acalculia, or loss of order and position of digits, and (3) anarithmia (or anarithmetia, the inability to perform arithmetic operations). Anarithmia and alexia for numbers are more often observed in cases of left-hemisphere retrorolandic lesions while spatial acalculia is related to right-hemisphere damage. Other forms of acalculia have been mentioned in the literature (e.g., Grewel, 1960, wrote about frontal acalculia). Some authors believe the acalculia associated with Gerstmann's syndrome corresponds to anarithmia (Boller & Grafman, 1985). Anarithmia is a consequence of the loss of understanding of the hierarchic structure of numbers, of mathematical relations, and of the meaning of mathematical signs.

The distinction between alexia and agraphia for numbers and anarithmia, although conceptually valid, is sometimes difficult to establish in practice. Damage topography is similar in both (Levin & Spiers, 1985), and if the existence of Gerstmann's syndrome is accepted, it must be supposed that anarithmia is associated, at least to a certain degree, to agraphia. Deloche and Seron (1984, 1987) emphasized the existence of a double code (alphabetic and numerical) in calculation. Using transcoding tasks between both processes, they observed the presence of errors due to position in series, lexical errors (78; 130) in patients with Wernicke's aphasia. In Broca's aphasia, the problems are stack errors (15 vs. 50; 140 vs. 104) and, consequently, syntactic errors. In patients with Wernicke's aphasia, the error is more of a semantic type, and the deficits in calculations could be related to lexical semantic errors in the reading and writing of numbers.

Boller and Grafman (1983, 1985) considered that the ability to calculate could be altered in various ways as a result of (1) the inability to appreciate the meaning of the names of the numbers, (2) visuospatial deficits that interfere with the spatial arrangement of the numbers and also with the mechanical aspects of the operations, (3) inability to remember mathematical facts and to use them appropriately, and (4) defects in mathematical thinking and in the comprehension of the underlying operations. Perhaps, the inability to conceptualize quantities (numeracy) and to reverse operations (e.g., from addition to subtraction) could be added as well. Angular acalculia in Gerstmann's syndrome would correspond more to the aforementioned second and fourth defects, frequently associated with calculation disorders of the first type (alexic and agraphic acalculia) in Hecaen and associates' classificatory scheme. Table 2.25 presents a general classification of acalculia.

Arithmetical calculation is a complex accomplishment; as such, it is likely to comprise many subcomponents. The study of arithmetical difficulties in normal subjects, as in brain-damaged patients, can be extremely informative with respect to the structure of normal calculation systems. However, calculation test batteries particularly designed for neuropsychological purposes are not readily available.

The Spanish lexicon for representing quantities resembles the

TABLE 2.25   Types of Acalculia

Anarithmetia	Alexic acalculia
Aphasic acalculia	In central alexia
In Broca's aphasia	In alexia without agraphia
In Wernicke's aphasia	Agraphic acalculia
In conduction aphasia	Frontal acalculia
	Spatial acalculia

one used in English with only slight differences. The names of numbers from 11 to 15 are formed with a single lexical unit composed of a root that refers to the base number (1, 2, 3, 4, 5) plus the suffix -ce (i.e., *once, doce, trece, catorce, quince*). From 16 to 19 the numbers are as follows: ten and six, ten and seven, ten and eight, and ten and nine (*dieciseis, diecisiete, dieciocho, diecinueve*). The number 20 (*veinte*) has no apparent relation to the number 2 (*dos*). The numbers 30, 40, 50, 60, 70, 80, and 90 are formed by a root referring to the base number plus the suffix -enta (*treinta, cuarenta, cincuenta, sesenta, setenta, ochenta, noventa*). The numbers 21–29, 31–39, and so on, are formed as twenty and one, twenty and two, and so forth. In Spanish, twenty and one would be *veintiuno*, etc. The word for 100 is *cien*, with no apparent relation to the number one (*uno*). After 100 the names of numbers become *ciento* plus the other number (*ciento uno, ciento dos*, etc.). For hundreds up to 900 the quantities are expressed as single words: two hundreds (*doscientos*), three hundreds (*trescientos*), and so on. The numbers from 21 to 29 can be written as a single word as well (*veintiuno, veintidos*, etc.). Sometimes the numbers 16 to 19 are written as a single word as well. The word for 1000 is *mil*. For quantities greater than 1000, the expression is *mil* (with no plural) plus the other number; for example, 2437 is *dos mil cuatrocientos treinta y siete*.

Testing Procedure

A battery for testing arithmetical abilities (see Appendix A11) was designed and includes the following sections:

1. Reading of numbers
2. Writing of numbers
3. Transcoding from numbers to letters
4. Transcoding from letters to numbers
5. Relationships "greater than" and "smaller than"
6. Mental arithmetical operations
7. Written arithmetical operations
8. Complex written arithmetical operations
9. Reading of arithmetical signs
10. Successive operations
11. Forward and backward counting
12. Aligning numbers in columns
13. Word problems

Normative Data

The Calculation Ability Test was given to 180 neurologically normal adults divided into three educational groups (0–5, 6–12, and more than 12 years of formal education) and three age ranges (16–30, 31–50, and 51–65 years). Statistically significant differences according to the educational level were found ($F = 22.98$; $df = 2$; $p<.001$). Weaker statistical differences according to age groups ($F = 3.57$; $df = 2$; $p<.05$) and sex ($F = 4.691$; $df = 1$; $p<.05$) were observed. No interaction was significant. Average number of errors were 12.92, 8.05 and 4.70 in the three analyzed educational levels. Average number of errors for the three age ranges were 10.43, 7.70 and 7.53. Average number of errors were 7.48 and 9.63 for males and females, respectively. A correction score according to the educational level is proposed (see Table 2.26).

Results in Brain-Damaged Patients

The Calculation Ability Test was given to 64 brain-damaged patients, 42 with left-hemisphere damage and 22 with right-hemisphere damage (Rosselli & Ardila, 1989). Comparisons between normal subjects and brain-damaged subjects showed significant differences for all subtests (except for the counting-forward subtest, in which there was no difference between normals and the right-hemisphere group). Differences between scores for patients with left- compared to right-hemisphere lesions were significant for the following subtests: reading numbers, reading arithmetical signs, successive operations, and backward counting. Score differences between patients with pre- and retrorolandic lesions in the left hemisphere were significant for transcoding (verbal to numerical and numerical to verbal), for complex

TABLE 2.26. Correction Score According to Educational Level for the Calculation Ability Test

Years of education	Correction scores
<6 years	−13
6–12 years	−9
>12 years	−5

arithmetic operations, and successive operations. In most cases the retrorolandic group presented a higher number of errors.

Test results for subgroups of patients with different left-hemisphere damage were analyzed. Transcoding from numerical to verbal code was a particularly difficult task for all patient subgroups, except for fluent aphasics; transcoding from verbal to numerical code was equally difficult for all patients, except patients with prefrontal damage. Utmost impairment in reading and writing numbers was found in patients with Broca's and conduction aphasia. Reading arithmetical signs was particularly difficult for fluent aphasics.

In most groups a higher incidence of errors was registered for the counting backwards subtest. In Broca's aphasia patients, counting in general was very difficult due to impairment in the oral production of language. Conduction aphasics presented a very clear dissociation in counting forward and backward, revealing omissions and substitutions. In patients with Wernicke's aphasia, omissions and substitutions were also observed with displacement of the series (e.g., 71, 72, 73, 85, 86 . . .). Lexical substitutions were frequent for all the groups in the counting backward subtest while some patients made lexical and syntactical number substitutions and lost the series completely.

Complex arithmetical operations, mental operations, and written operations were, in general, difficult for all brain-damaged patients. Those with Wernicke's aphasia had the highest number of errors in complex arithmetical operations and, compared with the rest of the groups, the least impairment in the word problems subtest; conduction aphasics displayed the largest number of errors in the latter subtest.

Different types of errors were analyzed. Decomposition errors in reading numbers (e.g., reading 125 as twelve five) hierarchy errors (e.g., misreading 5 as 50) and order errors (misreading 5 as 6) were evident in patients with Wernicke's and conduction aphasia. Inversions (e.g., reading 23 as 32) were more frequent in the anomic group, and perseverations were evident in patients with left prefrontal damage. The right-hemisphere group presented inversions and omission errors, the latter due to neglect.

In the complex arithmetic operations subtests the ability to carry appeared as the most frequent mistake. Patients with anomia and Wernicke's aphasia presented errors in the identification of arithmetical signs, and it was mainly the latter patients who, besides having difficulties in carrying, mixed procedures. Patients with right-hemisphere lesions also showed deficits in carrying (their difficulty being that they did not know where to put the carried quantity) and mixed procedures. Reasoning mistakes were also observed in these patients. For instance, they failed to recognize the absurdity of obtaining a larger number in a subtraction problem than the number being subtracted from. Blatant difficulties in aligning numbers in columns were also observed. It is important to note that many right-hemisphere patients had severe difficulty remembering the multiplication tables.

Various studies have analyzed the performance of brain-damaged patients on calculation tasks. Dahmen, Hartje, Bussing, and Strum (1982) studied calculation disorders in patients with Broca's and Wernicke's aphasia. Using factor analysis, they were able to identify two different factors: numeric-symbolic and visuospatial. The less severe calculation defects found in patients with Broca's aphasia are derived from their linguistic alterations while those found in patients with Wernicke's aphasia are due to aberrations in visuospatial processing. Jackson and Warrington (1986) compared the arithmetic skills of patients with left- and right-hemisphere damage and found significant differences between the two groups: the left-hemisphere lesion group showed greater impairment. However, the left-hemisphere lesion group was significantly more impaired in arithmetical computation than in arithmetical reasoning. Warrington (1982) demonstrated a dissociation between arithmetical processing in general and accurate retrieval of specific computation values. A selective deficit in processing operational signs—independent of the ability to understand numbers, retrieve arithmetic facts, and carry out calculation procedures—has been observed by Caramazza and McCloskey (1987) and Ferro and Botelho (1980). The dissociations described in these cases demonstrate different patterns of calculating deficits. Through analysis of the patterns of impaired performance in single-case studies (e.g., Benson & Denckla, 1969; Caramazza & McCloskey, 1987; Ferro & Botelho, 1980; McCloskey & Caramazza, 1987; Warrington, 1982) understanding of the cognitive processes of arithmetical calculation has been enhanced and models of normal number processing have been developed.

Chapter 3

Memory

WECHSLER MEMORY SCALE

Background

The most frequently used memory battery in clinical neuropsychology is the Wechsler Memory Scale (WMS), developed by Wechsler in 1945 and recently revised. The original test has two parallel forms (Form I and Form II), but Form I is more commonly used and has been studied more. The two forms have sufficient parallel-form reliability to be clinically interchangeable. WMS was designed to obtain a memory quotient (MQ) similar to the intelligence quotient (IQ). An MQ 12 points below the IQ has been suggested as an indication of memory impairment (Prigatano, 1978). Factor analysis has disclosed the existence of three different factors loading the WMS: (1) short-term verbal learning, (2) attention/concentration, and (3) orientation (Larrebee, Kane, & Schunck, 1983).

In 1975 Russell proposed using only the Logical Memory and Visual Reproduction subtests, which provide a balanced assessment of verbal (semantic memory) and nonverbal memory (configural memory). The subtests are administered in the traditional way, but a delayed recall is introduced after about half an hour. This new procedure allows calculation of three scores: (1) immediate recall, (2) delayed recall, and (3) percent retained (delayed recall divided by immediate recall and multiplied by 100). This modified procedure correlates well with other measures of brain dysfunction and can be used effectively to discriminate between normal elderly and demented subjects (Logue & Wyrick, 1979). Normative data for the WMS have been developed for normal subjects, brain-damaged patients (Russell, 1975, 1988), elderly populations (Halland, Linn, Hunt, & Goodwin,

1983; Margolis & Scialfa, 1984), and children (Curry, Logue, & Butler, 1986). Zagar, Arbit, Stuckey, and Wengel (1984) showed that the WMS subtests most sensitive to the effects of age are visuospatial memory tasks, remembering stories, and learning pairs of associated words.

During the 1970s a revision of the WMS battery was undertaken; it was completed and published in 1987 (Wechsler, 1987). The initial normalization sample of the WMS included about 200 subjects. Several normalization studies have been conducted (for a review of normative studies, see D'Elia, Satz, & Schretlen, 1989; Wallace, 1984). The majority of these studies, however, have not analyzed the influence of educational level on performance.

Test Description

The WMS is composed of the following seven sections:

    I.   Personal Information
   II.   Orientation
  III.   Mental Control
  IV.   Logical Memory
   V.   Digit Span
  VI.   Visual Reproduction
 VII.   Associative Learning

Sections I and II are composed of 6 and 5 items, respectively; each item is scored either 1 (correct) or 0 (incorrect). Section III is made of three items (counting backward from 20, reciting the alphabet, and counting by 3's from 1); the score for each item is 3 points if there are no errors within 10, 10, and 20 seconds, respectively; 2 points if there are no errors within the limit time (30, 30, and 45 seconds); and 1 point for only one error. In Section IV, which consists of two paragraphs with a total of 46 ideas, each idea recalled is scored 1; the final score is the average for both paragraphs (maximum score is 23). Digit Span (Section V) is made of lists of digits to be repeated forward and backward; the score is the maximum number of digits repeated in the correct order, forward plus backward (maximum score is 15). Section VI (Visual Reproduction) includes three cards with designs (Figure 3.1). Each card is presented to the subject for 10 seconds; immediately after the card has been removed from sight, the subject is instructed to draw the design from memory. Each design is scored separately, and all three scores are then summed to obtain a total Visual Reproduction score (maximum total score is 14). The Associate Learning subtest (Section VII) includes ten pairs of words; after read-

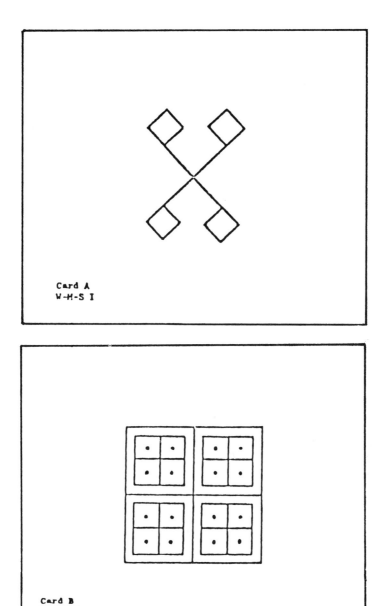

Card A
W-M-S I

Card B
W-M-S I

FIGURE 3.1

ing the words to the subject, the examiner then reads the first word of each pair, and the subject is asked to recall the paired word. The series is presented up to three times. Some associations are considered easy, others difficult. For each correct easy pair, $\frac{1}{2}$ point is earned, for each correct difficult pair 1 point, the maximum total score being 21.

The raw scores for all the sections are summed to obtain a Memory Quotient (MQ), which includes a correction score for the subject's age. In a large population, a mean of 100 and a standard deviation of 15 is expected.

The Spanish version of the WMS is available from the Psychological Corporation, 555 Academic Court, San Antonio, TX 78204; 1-800-228-0752.

Normative Data

The Spanish version of the WMS Form I was given to 300 neurologically normal subjects. A brief neurological and psychiatric screening was administered to verify existing information about the subjects; all subjects performed adequately in everyday activities. Subjects were divided according to age (20–29, 30–39, 40–49, 50–59, and 60–69 years), sex, and educational level (0–5, 6–12, and more than 12 years of formal education). A 5 × 2 × 3 design with 10 subjects in each cell was developed. The mean scores and the standard deviations for each section of the WMS are presented in Tables 3.1 (Information), 3.2 (Orientation), 3.3 (Mental Control), 3.4 (Digit Span), 3.5 (Logical Memory), 3.6 (Visual Reproduction) and 3.7 (Associate Learning).

TABLE 3.1. Mean Scores (and Standard Deviations) of Normal Subjects on the Information Subtest of the Wechsler Memory Scale ($N = 300$)

| Education | Age (years) | | | | | |
	20–29	30–39	40–49	50–59	60–69	Average
0–5 years	4.74	4.80	4.65	4.58	4.50	4.65
	(1.25)	(1.17)	(1.06)	(1.39)	(0.84)	(1.14)
6–12 years	5.30	5.25	5.25	5.21	5.25	5.25
	(0.56)	(0.77)	(1.21)	(0.57)	(0.90)	(0.80)
>12 years	5.40	5.55	5.25	5.55	5.50	5.45
	(0.65)	(0.59)	(0.77)	(0.60)	(1.04)	(0.73)
Average	5.15	5.20	5.05	5.11	5.08	5.11
	(0.82)	(0.84)	(1.01)	(0.85)	(0.92)	(0.89)

TABLE 3.2. Mean Scores (and Standard Deviations)
of Normal Subjects on the Orientation Subtest
of the Wechsler Memory Scale (N = 300)

Education	Age (years)					
	20–29	30–39	40–49	50–59	60–69	Average
0–5 years	4.89	4.85	4.85	4.71	4.70	4.80
	(0.31)	(0.57)	(0.36)	(0.55)	(0.56)	(0.47)
6–12 years	4.80	4.84	4.95	4.85	4.76	4.84
	(0.50)	(0.36)	(0.21)	(0.35)	(0.42)	(0.37)
>12 years	4.95	5.00	4.90	4.89	5.00	4.95
	(0.15)	(0.00)	(0.30)	(0.46)	(0.00)	(0.18)
Average	4.88	4.89	4.90	4.82	4.82	4.80
	(0.32)	(0.31)	(0.29)	(0.45)	(0.33)	(0.34)

The influence of the subject's age and, particularly, educational level was statistically significant for most of the subtests; therefore, a score correction of the total raw score is suggested (see Table 3.8); this correction score should be added to the subject's total raw score before the MQ is obtained (Wechsler, 1945).

Results in Brain-Damaged Populations

The WMS has been extensively used in the clinical analysis of brain-damaged populations. Selected recent studies in clinical neuropsychology using the WMS are briefly presented here.

TABLE 3.3. Mean Scores (and Standard Deviations)
of Normal Subjects on the Mental Control Subtest
of the Wechsler Memory Scale (N = 300)

Education	Age (years)					
	20–29	30–39	40–49	50–59	60–69	Average
0–5 years	4.16	4.00	3.50	3.90	3.70	3.85
	(1.95)	(1.90)	(1.96)	(1.80)	(0.65)	(1.85)
6–12 years	4.95	4.85	4.45	4.55	4.68	4.69
	(2.52)	(2.43)	(2.59)	(2.25)	(1.15)	(2.19)
>12 years	6.40	5.95	4.49	6.06	6.00	4.63
	(2.40)	(1.62)	(2.12)	(2.14)	(2.22)	(2.10)
Average	5.17	4.93	4.15	4.84	4.79	4.39
	(2.29)	(1.98)	(2.22)	(2.06)	(1.67)	(2.05)

TABLE 3.4.   Mean Scores (and Standard Deviations)
of Normal Subjects on the Digit Span Subtest
of the Wechsler Memory Scale (N = 300)

Education	Age (years)					
	20–29	30–39	40–49	50–59	60–69	Average
0–5 years	8.11	8.05	7.95	7.90	7.82	7.98
	(1.16)	(1.28)	(0.74)	(1.20)	(1.30)	(1.14)
6–12 years	9.05	8.58	8.75	8.35	8.06	8.56
	(2.22)	(1.31)	(1.33)	(1.27)	(0.74)	(1.37)
>12 years	10.50	9.95	9.40	9.11	9.02	9.60
	(1.50)	(1.71)	(1.24)	(1.82)	(1.04)	(1.46)
Average	9.22	8.86	8.70	8.45	8.30	8.71
	(1.63)	(1.43)	(1.10)	(1.43)	(1.03)	(1.32)

Coorigan and Hinkeldey (1987) administered the WMS to a
rehabilitation population suffering from unilateral cerebrovascular
accidents and closed-head injury. Results showed that poorer memory scores were observed in patients with head injury and diffuse
brain damage than normal. Alekoumbides, Charter, Adkins, and Seacat (1987) were able to construct differential WMS profiles for patients with focal brain damage, Korsakoff's syndrome, and dementia.
Hightower and Anderson (1986) used Russell's revision of the WMS
with alcoholic patients; although differences according to abuse

TABLE 3.5.   Mean Scores (and Standard Deviations)
of Normal Subjects on the Logical Memory Subtest
of the Wechsler Memory Scale (N = 300)

Education	Age (years)					
	20–29	30–39	40–49	50–59	60–69	Average
0–5 years	11.13	12.41	11.56	10.34	9.96	11.08
	(3.76)	(3.19)	(3.02)	(3.38)	(3.43)	(3.35)
6–12 years	13.43	12.12	13.09	11.85	10.21	12.14
	(3.69)	(3.03)	(4.35)	(2.28)	(1.88)	(3.04)
>12 years	17.12	17.35	15.97	13.69	12.89	15.40
	(3.19)	(3.20)	(3.40)	(3.67)	(3.71)	(3.79)
Average	13.89	13.96	13.54	11.96	11.02	12.87
	(3.55)	(3.21)	(3.68)	(3.12)	(3.03)	(3.31)

TABLE 3.6. Mean Scores (and Standard Deviations)
of Normal Subjects on the Visual Reproduction Subtest
of the Wechsler Memory Scale (N = 300)

Education	Age (years)					
	20–29	30–39	40–49	50–59	60–69	Average
0–5 years	7.47	6.70	6.35	6.05	3.40	5.99
	(3.45)	(2.74)	(3.78)	(3.85)	(2.85)	(3.33)
6–12 years	8.25	8.15	8.15	6.50	5.75	7.36
	(2.70)	(3.49)	(3.21)	(2.64)	(1.85)	(2.79)
>12 years	10.40	9.45	9.45	8.12	7.13	8.91
	(1.75)	(2.52)	(2.25)	(3.71)	(1.99)	(2.23)
Average	8.71	8.10	7.98	6.89	5.42	7.42
	(2.63)	(2.92)	(3.08)	(3.40)	(2.23)	(2.85)

status and age were found, alcoholics demonstrated only mild deficits when compared with age-matched controls.

Botwinick, Storandt, and Berg (1986) compared the performance of normal healthy adults and patients with Alzheimer's disease during a period of 4 years. Normal subjects showed little decline in performance on the WMS over the 4-year period, while patients with dementia showed a progressive decline on all subtests. The largest declines were seen with the Logical Memory subtest, the smallest with the Digit Span forward subtest. The WMS has also been used

TABLE 3.7. Mean Scores (and Standard Deviations)
of Normal Subjects on the Associative Learning Subtest
of the Wechsler Memory Scale (N = 300)

Education	Age (years)					
	20–29	30–39	40–49	50–59	60–69	Average
0–5 years	13.18	14.90	14.45	13.27	11.20	13.40
	(2.97)	(2.94)	(3.18)	(4.87)	(3.78)	(3.55)
6–12 years	15.60	15.20	14.90	14.47	13.31	14.70
	(3.35)	(2.52)	(3.59)	(1.89)	(3.10)	(2.89)
>12 years	18.20	17.42	16.80	16.28	16.26	17.01
	(1.25)	(2.00)	(3.07)	(2.33)	(3.19)	(2.37)
Average	15.66	15.87	15.55	14.67	13.59	15.04
	(2.52)	(2.50)	(3.28)	(3.03)	(3.36)	(2.94)

TABLE 3.8.   Score Correction
of the Wechsler Memory Scale Raw Score
for Age and Educational Attainment

Education	Age (years)				
	20–29	30–39	40–49	50–59	60–69
0–5 years	44	45	46	49	55
6–12 years	39	41	42	44	48
>12 years	30	32	34	36	37

Note. The correction score is added to the total raw score.

to study dementia associated with Huntington's disease (Brandt, 1984).

VERBAL SERIAL LEARNING CURVE

Background

The process of memorizing and recalling information involves three phases: imprinting, or reception of the information; storing, or conservation of the information; and recall, or reproduction of the stored material (Luria, 1966; Ardila, 1986). Disturbances of the memory process due to lesions in different parts of the brain have been observed. Hence, a primary aim of the neuropsychological assessment of memory is to establish which aspect of the memory process is being disturbed.

One of the most popular procedures for the evaluation of verbal memory is the Serial Learning Test (e.g., D'Amato, 1970), in which the subject is presented with a series of verbal elements (syllables, numbers, and words) that are to be learned over the course of several trials. Using this test, the clinician is able to determine the limits of subjects' ability to memorize, as well as characteristics of the process of verbal learning. Luria (1966, 1975, 1976b) adapted and extensively used this particular procedure in neuropsychological assessment. Luria's adaptation of the serial learning test consists of the successive presentation of a series of words (usually, but not necessarily, 10). Once the words are read, the subject tries to recall as many of them as possible. The entire list of words is repeated over and over again until the subject can recall all the words on the list. The order of recalling the words is not important; what is relevant is the number of words recalled in each trial. In normal subjects, usually no more than 10 presentations are required to obtain complete recall. According to Luria, this test represents one of the most powerful and informative memory tests. Short-term memory span, decreases in verbal learning, confabulations, intrusions, perseverations, and attentional deficits are readily observed. Frequently, delayed recall is also included as part of the test. Numerous examples of pathological performance on this test have been analyzed by Luria (1966, 1976b).

Luria (1976b) reported limited normative data for the serial learning test. He predicted that a normal person would recall about five or six words out of ten after a single presentation and that about four presentations of the series are required for successfully recalling all ten words. In normal populations a positively increasing curve is always observed. However, age and educational level should be taken into consideration since these variables affect the learning curve.

Test Description

Ten bisyllabic high-frequency Spanish (or ten monosyllabic English) nouns were selected (see Appendix A12). A list of words was read to the subject at a rate of one word per second after the following instructions: "I am going to read you a series of very simple words; when I finish, I want you to say all the words you can recall, in any order." Once the list is read, the subject immediately tries to recall the words. On the test sheet the examiner writes down (below each word and in a line designated for the first trial) the word recall order (1, 2, 3, . . .). When the subject finishes saying the words, the examiner reads the same list again after the following instructions: "Now I am going to read the same list again, and I want you to say in any order all the words you can remember; it does not matter if you have said them in the former trial." The examiner records the word recall order again on the test sheet, this time using the line corresponding to the second trial. Using the same instructions used in the second presentation, the examiner continues to read the entire list to the subject (up to 10 times) until the subject is able to learn all 10 words. In every trial the subject tries to repeat all the words; it is critical if a forgotten word has already been retrieved in a previous trial. If the subject is unable to retrieve the 10 words after 10 presentations, the test is discontinued. The examiner writes down the order of the recalled words for each trial and also takes note of all mistakes, such as intrusions (words not belonging to the series) and perseverations (repetition of the same word in one particular trial). In order to test delayed verbal memory, subjects are asked to recall the words of the list after a delay of 10 to 15 minutes.

Scoring

Once completed, the examiner scores the results by counting the number of words in each trial and the number of trials required for learning the 10 words. The number of words recalled in the first trial is the subject's immediate verbal memory. A score lower than 4 may be considered abnormal, but a subject's age and educational level should be considered. The results of each trial can be plotted to yield a subject's learning curve. The number of words are indicated on the vertical axis, the number of trials on the horizontal axis. A "productive" curve means that there is an improvement from trial to trial; a "nonproductive" curve reaches a certain maximum level on the first trial and remains the same (or even decreases); "stereotyped" curve means that the same words are reproduced trial after trial with little change; and a "disorganized" curve suggests that different words are retrieved in each trial but without an accumulative gain. The number of words recalled in delayed memory is also plotted on the curve. It is estimated that normal subjects recall six or seven words 10 to 15 minutes after the last presentation. The interpretation of delayed verbal memory also depends on the subject's age and level of education.

Besides the learning curve, other types of information about the subject's performance should be recorded. This would include (1) recall order in each trial, (2) the number of trials, and (3) the number of intrusions. The cognitive strategy used by the subject can usually be analyzed from the recall order. For example, normal subjects usually start a new trial (after the first one) by first saying the words they have not said before (and that are more sensitive to forgetfulness), followed by the words they have said in previous trials (and that are already learned). This strategy may help the subject show an improvement on the learning curve. Brain-damaged patients, in contrast, may lack any cognitive strategy and may offer the same sequence of words over trials. In the number of trials required to learn the 10 words, it is estimated that normal subjects require from five to ten trials, depending on the subject's age and level of education. If after ten trials the subject is unable to learn the 10 words, the examiner writes down the number of words recalled in the last trial. This number of words is the patient's peak score of verbal learning. Finally, the number of intrusions (words not included in the list) and perseverations (number of times a word is repeated in one trial) and the types of errors observed may be important in integrating the results of the neuropsychological assessment. The volume of retained material increases during learning and the subject's reaction (indifference, concern, etc.) to mistakes made is important in the interpretation of the test results. In the recall of words in delayed memory, a "reminiscence" (i.e., recall of a word that was not said during the learning process) is occasionally observed. This seems to appear frequently in the normal population.

Normative Data

The test was administered to two different samples: sample A consisted of 180 Spanish-speaking subjects (90 males and 90 females) belonging to three different education levels (0–5, 6–12, and more than 12 years of education) and within the age range of 16 to 65 years; sample B was composed of 326 Spanish-speaking subjects (163 females and 163 males) belonging to three different educational groups (0–5, 6–12, and more than 12 years of education) and within the age range of 56 to 80 years. All subjects were healthy persons, performing adequately in everyday life activities and without a history of psychiatric or neurological disorders.

Table 3.9 shows the means and standard deviations of subjects'

TABLE 3.9. Means (and Standard Deviations) According to Age and Level of Education for Words Recalled by Normal Subjects in a First Trial (Verbal Serial Learning Curve) ($N = 326$)

Age (years)	Education (years)			Age (years)	Education (years)		
	0–5	6–12	>12		0–5	6–12	>12
16–30	5.60	6.37	6.67	66–70	4.00	4.89	5.41
	(1.19)	(1.36)	(1.53)		(1.22)	(1.43)	(1.48)
31–50	5.28	5.65	6.18	71–75	3.85	4.23	5.00
	(1.07)	(1.09)	(2.53)		(1.19)	(1.38)	(1.40)
51–60	5.00	5.22	5.67	>76	3.68	4.09	4.30
	(1.33)	(2.56)	(1.85)		(1.22)	(1.42)	(1.37)
61–65	4.48	4.96	5.52				
	(1.20)	(1.54)	(1.53)				

scores for recalled words in a first trial, according to the subject's age and level of education, for the two samples studied. Observe that the memory span increases with educational level and decreases with age. There were no differences between males and females.

Table 3.10 shows the means and standard deviations of the number of trials required for subjects to successfully recall the ten words. Note that some subjects (particularly older ones with lower educational levels) could not retrieve the ten words even after 10 presentations. However, they could usually recall nine (and, in isolated cases, just eight) words. Those subjects who were unable to learn the list of words after 10 trials received a score of 11. This performance was frequently observed in the oldest group (older than 76 years) with the lowest level of education (0 to 5 years). In general, the number of trials increased with the subject's age and decreased with educational level. It is worth mentioning that occasionally a subject recalled all ten words after a single presentation, but this was rare. In some subjects the number of words recalled increased up to a certain point and then, in further presentations, either decreased or remained the same, yielding a plateau-like curve; the decrement may be interpreted as the result of fatigue and was particularly true of the learning curve for older subjects.

Results of the delayed recall measure disclosed a very mild forgetfulness of the words in the youngest groups, with subjects forgetting only one to two words, on average, after some 10 to 15

TABLE 3.10. Means (and Standard Deviations)
According to Age and Level of Education for the Number
of Trials by Normal Subjects for Recalling Ten Words
(Verbal Serial Learning Curve; $N = 526$)

Age (years)	Education (years)			Age (years)	Education (years)		
	0–5	6–12	>12		0–5	6–12	>12
16–30	6.30	5.06	5.00	66–70	9.75	8.45	7.52
	(2.81)	(3.19)	(2.65)		(2.50)	(2.35)	(2.42)
31–50	6.33	6.20	5.14	71–75	9.90	8.92	7.57
	(2.59)	(2.65)	(2.51)		(2.63)	(2.71)	(2.74)
51–60	7.89	6.61	6.53	>76	10.14	9.00	7.86
	(2.10)	(3.06)	(3.01)		(3.02)	(3.04)	(3.08)
61–65	9.05	7.89	7.24				
	(2.20)	(2.25)	(2.30)				

minutes. However, in the oldest and less educated groups, the score for delayed memory decreased to five words (see Table 3.11).

Using only the scores obtained by subjects of sample B (N = 346) a normalization of raw scores was completed (see Appendix B, Table B5). Standard scores (percentages, percentiles, and T scores) are presented for the following four age and educational groups: age 55–65 years and 0–5 years of formal education; age 55–65 years and more than 5 years of formal education; age 66 years and over and 0–5 years of formal education; and age 55 years and over and an educational level of more than 5 years of formal education. Groups were divided in this manner after determining that the major score differences were found between these age groups and educational levels.

Results in Brain-Damaged Patients

Most of the clinical research on the use of this memory test with neurologically impaired subjects has been carried out by Luria (1966, 1975, 1976b). Different types of learning curves and different patterns of errors have been associated with specific brain pathology. For example, nonproductive stereotyped curves with perseveration are observed in frontal lobe patients. These subjects memorize a few words (usually no more than three) in one presentation and on the following presentations continue to repeat the same words as before without comparing their result with the original series. Patients with

TABLE 3.11. Means (and Standard Deviations) According to Age and Level of Education for the Delayed Recall (10–15 minutes) of Ten Words for Normal Subjects (Verbal Serial Learning Curve; N = 526)

Age (years)	Education (years)			Age (years)	Education (years)		
	0–5	6–12	>12		0–5	6–12	>12
16–30	9.02	9.10	9.11	66–70	6.32	7.42	7.77
	(0.95)	(1.47)	(0.67)		(1.59)	(1.62)	(1.48)
31–50	8.33	8.64	8.70	71–75	6.21	7.05	6.35
	(1.53)	(1.17)	(1.89)		(1.61)	(1.65)	(1.69)
51–60	7.50	8.15	8.22	>76	4.95	5.91	7.33
	(1.57)	(1.17)	(1.89)		(1.61)	(1.53)	(1.49)
61–65	7.19	7.75	7.81				
	(1.52)	(1.47)	(1.63)				

frontal lobe damage may present learning curves that increase up to a certain point and afterward plateau or fluctuate but always remain at a low level of performance. For example, in successive trials the patient may recall four, five, six, five, and four words. Patients with frontal lobe damage are usually unaware of mistakes (i.e., there is no error awareness) and cannot correct an incorrectly reproduced series (i.e., there is no error utilization). Indeed, they consistently repeat the same mistakes as they exhibit the lack of a cognitive strategy. According to Luria, when normal people are preparing to learn a list of words, they set a goal establishing the number of words they anticipate learning on each trial. Usually, this level of expectation is higher than the subject's actual performance. Frontal lobe patients do not establish a goal and do not make a strategy to improve their performance. Confabulation is routinely observed in frontal lobe patients, particularly in those with orbit area damage and in those with general head trauma. Further, intrusions are readily observed in frontal lobe damage.

Patients with posterior brain lesions (but not aphasics) show a learning process similar to that of normal subjects. They establish a goal level, correct their mistakes, and produce rising learning curves. Compared to normal subjects, the patient's learning curve rises more slowly, the volume of material learned is smaller (the peak of the curve is no higher than six words), and there is a tendency to experience fatigue more easily during the learning process.

Korsakoff's syndrome is associated with nonproductive and disorganized verbal learning curves; frequently, the patient presents intrusions related to a confabulatory tendency. Hippocampal amnesia is associated with nonproductive curves without intrusions. In both types of amnesia the delayed recall of words is not expected.

In Alzheimer's disease, selective memory deficits are often the first neuropsychological finding. When performing a verbal serial learning test, Alzheimer's disease patients show perseveration, a lack of encoding strategies, and a higher degree of vulnerability to interference, as compared to elderly subjects who do not have the disease (Albert & Moss, 1984). The recalling of words over time is particularly impaired. Weingartner, Kaye, and Smalling (1982) reported that Alzheimer's disease patients were unable to use the semantics of words as a strategy for encoding the learning material.

Other important information that can be obtained from the first trial of the verbal learning test has to do with the serial position effect: the words presented in the first few positions (the primacy effect) and those presented in the last few positions (the recency effect) are favored in recall over those in the middle of the list. Patients with Alzheimer's disease tend to exhibit the recency effect but not the primacy effect (Miller, 1977). This might be due to an increased sensitivity to interference.

The verbal serial learning task has been shown to be one of the most sensitive to the effects of aging (Ardila & Rosselli, 1989). The second most important factor underlying cognitive changes was represented by the verbal learning test in aging found in a factor analysis of the results of a neuropsychological battery given to elderly subjects. Using a correction score for age avoids false positive results in the elderly, i.e., labeling/including a normal person as brain-damaged.

DIGIT SPAN TEST

Background

The time interval involved in different types of memory processes ranges from fractions of a second in sensorial memory to years in long-term memory. Of special interest to neuropsychologists is immediate memory, which refers to information retained several seconds after a single presentation.

Digit Span has been considered the fundamental test in measuring immediate memory (Lezak, 1983). Traditionally, it is included in several psychological and neuropsychological test batteries, such as the Wechsler Adult Intelligence Scale (1955), the Stanford-Binet Intelligence Scale (Terman & Merrill, 1973), the Wechsler Memory Scale (Wechsler, 1945), and the revised versions of the Wechsler tests.

Digit Span usually includes two parts: Digits Forward and Digits Backward, with various procedures. The Wechsler Intelligence Scale subtest includes seven pairs of random number sequences. In the Wechsler Memory Scale, Digits Forward involves five pairs of sequenced numbers, the sequences ranging from four to eight digits; Digits Backward involves five pairs, with sequences ranging from three to seven digits. The examiner reads the digits aloud at a rate of one per second. In the Digits Backward subtest, the subject is required to repeat the digits in the exact reverse order. In both cases the test is interrupted when the subject fails to repeat two consecutive sets of digits. However, variations of these procedures are also used. For instance, Lezak (1983) suggests giving a third sequence of the same length when the subject's failure may be due to distraction or noncooperation. When subjects do better on Digits Backward than Digits Forward, it can be suspected that they are capable of doing at least as well on the latter. Some clinicians prefer presenting a series of digits increasing in number, interrupting only after the subject fails on two consecutive trials.

The order of the digits recalled is an important variable. However, when a subject correctly recalls the digits of a series but fails to recall the correct order, a certain level of immediate memory processing is taking place. Digits Forward measures auditory attention and immediate memory. Passive memory span is required. Digits Backward requires a mental reversal and, therefore, a working memory: a double tracking is required, since both memory and reversing operations must proceed simultaneously.

Normal performance in Digits Forward has been considered to be about 6 ± 1 (Spitz, 1972). In Digits Backward it is considered to be around 4 to 5 (Lezak, 1983). Normal differences between Digits Forward and Digits Backward can be between 1 (Costa, 1975) to 2 numbers (Black & Strub, 1978).

There are some studies reporting the effects of education on Digit Span (Weinberg, Diller, Gerstman, & Schulman, 1972). Subjects of higher educational attainment present a better performance on this task than do those with less education. Botwinick and Storandt (1974) have studied the effects of age on Digit Span performance: although Digits Forward is less sensitive to the effects of aging, Digits Backward typically decreases about one point during the seventh decade of life.

Normative Data

Digit Span was given to 346 subjects divided into groups according to age (56–60, 61–65, 66–70, 71–75, and more than 75 years), sex, and educational level (0–5, 6–12, and more than 12 years of formal education). Table 3.12 shows the F values for the three variables. Note that differences are statistically significant for educational groups, both for Digits Forward and for Digits Backward. Differences for age groups are statistically significant only for Digits Backward. However, for Digits Backward, differences among educational groups are greater than differences among age groups; in other words, educational level is a stronger variable than age within the age ranges analyzed.

Table 3.13 shows the average number of digits recalled for each one of the age and educational levels included. No change in Digits

TABLE 3.12. F Values for the Digits Forward
and Digits Backward Subtests of Digit Span

	df	Mean square	f	Level of significance
Digits Forward				
Educational level (A)	2	41.498	45.872	0.001
Age (B)	4	2.239	2.475	NS
Sex (C)	1	0.015	0.016	NS
A × B	8	1.649	1.822	NS
A × C	2	0.019	0.021	NS
B × C	4	0.477	0.527	NS
A × B × C	8	0.528	0.584	NS
Digits Backward				
Educational level (A)	2	26.028	27.737	0.001
Age (B)	4	2.699	2.876	0.023
Sex (C)	1	0.956	1.019	NS
A × B	8	1.557	1.659	NS
A × C	2	0.929	0.990	NS
B × C	4	0.747	0.796	NS
A × B × C	8	0.711	0.758	NS

Forward across educational levels was observed. The lowest educational groups repeated an average of 4.5 for Digits Forward across all age groups while the highest educational groups repeated a score of 5.8. Therefore, there is a one-digit difference between the two extreme educational groups. In Digits Backward, performance is quite steady through the 71–75 years age range; in the oldest (more than 75 years) group there is a decrease of about 0.4 digits. The difference between performance on Digits Forward and Digits Backward was an average of 1.8 in the first four age ranges (from 56 to 75 years) and 2.2 for the oldest age group (more than 75 years). It is important to note that no sex differences were found: differences across ages and across educational levels were equivalent for males and females.

Norms (percentages, percentiles, and T scores) were obtained for the following four educational and age groups: age 55–65 years and 0–5 years of formal education; age 55–65 years and more than 5 years of formal education; over age 65 years and 0–5 years of formal education; and over age 65 years and more than 5 years of formal education. These norms are found in Appendix B, Table B6.

TABLE 3.13.   Digit Span Scores for Different Age Ranges
(N = 346)

Education (years)	Age (years)					
	56–60	61–65	66–70	71–75	>75	Mean
0–5						
Forward	4.5	4.5	4.5	4.5	4.5	4.5
Backward	2.9	2.9	2.8	2.8	2.7	2.8
6–12						
Forward	5.1	5.1	5.1	5.1	5.1	5.1
Backward	3.2	3.2	3.2	3.2	3.1	3.2
>12						
Forward	5.8	5.8	5.8	5.8	5.8	5.8
Backward	3.9	3.9	3.9	3.9	3.1	3.7
Mean						
Forward	5.1	5.1	5.1	5.1	5.1	5.1
Backward	3.3	3.3	3.3	3.3	2.9	3.2

Results in Brain-Damaged Patients

Digit Span is considered a sensitive test of brain damage, particularly left-hemisphere involvement (Weinberg et al., 1972). Patients with diffuse brain involvement present a decreased performance in digit retention, particularly in Digits Backward. Since this test is a measure of attention, people who have suffered brain injury show a decreased score. However, it has been reported that patients with Korsakoff's syndrome have a nearly normal performance on digit retention tests (Talland, 1965). Interestingly, patients with visual field defects have a shorter backward span than those without such defects (Lezak, 1983), most likely, the result of the inability to visualize information.

TEST OF MEMORY FOR UNFAMILIAR FACES

Background

Different procedures have been used to evaluate recognition and memory of faces. The most extensively used procedure has been the recognition of familiar faces. Lezak (1983) suggests that facial recognition tests can be divided into those that involve a memory component and those that do not. All tests of familiar faces imply recall of stored information since they test the ability to identify persons well known to the subject (Warrington & James, 1967).

Benton, Hamsher, Varney, and Spreen (1983) developed a test for the recognition of unfamiliar faces, that is, a test that limits memory involvement. The subject matches identical front views of unfamiliar faces, front views with side views, and front views taken under different lighting conditions.

The tests of unfamiliar faces involving memory include presenting a series of photographs to the subject, then they must match either one at a time or in sets of two or more a "new" set of photographs to the previous one. The subject is required to remember the distinguishing features of the faces in order to be able to match them. It is important to note that recognition and memory of faces are related to the familiarity of the facial type to the subject: it is well known that difficulty exists in identifying a face belonging to a member of a different racial group. Brain-damaged patients who have difficulty recognizing faces (prosopagnosia) also present difficulties in the identification of cars and animals and, in general, in distinguishing individual members of a specific visuoperceptual category.

Testing Procedure

A test was designed for assessing short-term memory for unfamiliar faces. The test includes 24 frontal photographs of young Caucasian men (see Appendix A13). Six of the photographs are repeated (those labeled with the following numbers: 9, 12, 15, 19, 22, and 24). Pictures are presented to the subject consecutively, with the following instruction: "I am going to show you some pictures of unknown people. Some of them are going to be repeated. I want you to tell me whenever you see a face that has been repeated." When the ninth photograph is shown, the subject is asked, "Please, let me know if this picture was presented before." The subject must answer yes or no. The examiner writes down the answer on the answer sheet (see Appendix A14). The maximum score (correct identification of previously presented faces) is 6 points. False positives must be registered.

Normative Data

The Test of Memory for Unfamiliar Faces was given to 346 neurologically intact subjects divided into groups according to age

(56–60, 61–65, 66–70, 71–75, and more than 75 years), sex, and educational level (0–5, 6–12, and more than 12 years of formal education). Table 3.14 shows the mean scores in the different age and educational groups. Differences among age groups ($F = 3.15$; $df = 4$; $p<.01$) and educational groups ($F = 6.77$; $df = 2$; $p<.001$) were statistically significant. However, differences between sexes were not significant ($F = 0.63$; $df = 1$; NS). No interactions were significant. The average correct recognition score was 5.04 (84%) for the youngest group analyzed and 4.23 (70%) for the oldest group. Differences according to educational level were observed only with regard to the group with the lowest educational level. The average correct recognition score (70%) for the group with 0–5 years of formal education group and for the oldest age group were the same. Differences between the group with 6–12 years of formal education and the group with more than 12 years of formal education were nonsignificant.

Norms (percentages, percentiles, and T scores) were obtained for the following four educational and age groups: age 55–65 years and 0–5 years of formal education; age 55–65 years and more than 5 years of formal education; over age 65 years and 0–5 years of formal education; and over age 65 years and more than 5 years of formal education (see Appendix B, Table B7).

Results in Brain-Damaged Populations

Studies involving the recognition of faces indicate that different brain mechanisms may underlie the recognition of familiar and unfamiliar faces. Face recognition of unfamiliar faces has been shown to be greater in right-hemisphere–damaged patients than in left (De

TABLE 3.14. Mean Scores (Correct Recognition Responses) for Normal Subjects on the Test of Memory for Unfamiliar Faces According to Age and Educational Level ($N = 346$)

Education (years)	Age (years)					
	55–60	61–65	66–70	71–75	>75	Average
0–5	4.91	4.50	4.10	3.80	3.77	4.22
6–12	5.25	4.79	4.59	4.86	4.52	4.80
>12	4.96	4.83	4.70	4.65	4.39	4.70
Average	5.04	4.71	4.46	4.44	4.23	4.57

Renzi, Faglioni, & Spinnler, 1968). De Renzi and Spinnler (1966) administered a test of face recognition to normal subjects and to those with damage to the left and right hemispheres of the brain. The subjects' task was to inspect a photograph of an unknown face for 15 seconds and to recognize the face from among 20 photographs of different faces immediately after the target photograph was removed. Normal subjects outperformed brain-damaged individuals, and left-hemisphere–damaged patients showed a superior performance over right-hemisphere–damaged individuals. Left-brain–damaged subjects hold a slight advantage over right-brain–damaged subjects in the immediate retrieval of schematic faces, a finding that was also reported by Murri, Arena, Siciliano, Mazzotta, and Muratorio (1984). Furthermore, retrorolandic-damaged subjects in the last-mentioned study showed the highest impairment. Support for the posterior involvement of the right hemisphere in facial recognition deficits has been repeatedly demonstrated in the literature (Bruyer, 1986). Milner (1968) showed that patients with right temporal involvement score lower than those with left temporal damage in an immediate face recognition task, and Warrington and James (1967) described a specific defect for face recognition in patients with right retrorolandic lesions.

In general, studies have affirmed that patients with right posterior (occipitotemporal) lesions have the greatest difficulty in performing recognition tasks involving unfamiliar faces. This group of patients shows impairment in the ability to store in memory previously unknown faces in order to recognize them in a subsequent trial (Bruyer, 1986). Poor performance of right-hemisphere–damaged subjects has also been shown in face discrimination tasks, that is, in tasks in which the subject does not need to keep information in memory but has only to match stimuli that are simultaneously presented. Evidence from the study of patients with prosopagnosia suggests that this type of visual agnosia is the result of bilateral lesions involving the occipitotemporal areas (Damasio, Damasio, & Van Hoesen, 1982; Damasio & Damasio, 1986). Consequently, it can be hypothesized that deficits in the recognition of familiar faces, or prosopagnosia, are usually the result of bilateral posterior hemispheric damage while deficits in memory for unfamiliar faces are associated with right occipitotemporal damage.

Chapter 4

Spatial and Praxic Abilities

REY-OSTERRIETH COMPLEX FIGURE TEST

Background

The Complex Figure Test was designed by Rey (1941) to assess visual perception and visual memory in brain-damaged subjects. In 1944, Osterrieth administered the Rey figure to 230 children ranging in age from 4 to 15 years old and to 60 adults between 16 and 60 years old (Lezak, 1983). In 1969, Taylor made an alternative figure to be used for retesting (Lezak, 1983). In contemporary neuropsychology, the Rey-Osterrieth Complex Figure is one of the most frequently used tests to assess constructional and visuospatial abilities.

The test consists of a design card showing a figure that contains 18 elements which could be scored (see Appendix A14). Subjects are asked to copy the figure, which is placed in front of them, on a white sheet of paper. The drawing sequence that the subject follows is registered in detail by the examiner. There are several methods of registering the subject's performance: In one method, the subject is given a different color each time he or she is going to start a different part of the figure, with the examiner writing down the color sequence used by the subject (Lezak, 1983). An alternate method of tracking the subject's performance is for the examiner to number another copy of the complex figure with the subject's drawing sequence. A much more difficult method of tracking the drawing sequence is for the examiner to reproduce simultaneously the performance of the subject, numbering each unit in the same order that it is being drawn (Lezak, 1983; Binder, 1982).

When the subject is finished copying the figure, both the design card and the subject's drawing are removed; the subject is then asked to draw the figure from memory, either immediately or after a delay. The recalled figure and the copied one are scored separately, with the maximum score being 36 (Taylor, 1959).

Normal adults achieve, on average, a score of 32 (Lezak, 1983). One of the two main procedures used in copying the design is to draw the large rectangle first and then add the details to it; the other procedure is to begin with a detail attached to the central rectangle or with a subsection of the central rectangle, complete the rectangle, and add remaining details in relation to the rectangle (Osterrieth, 1944; Lezak, 1983). Children older than 8 years of age score 30, on average, and from age 13 tend to follow the same procedures used by adults (Lezak, 1983). In children under 7, Waber and Holmes (1985) described a pattern of directionality (from right to left) in copying the Rey-Osterrieth Complex Figure. This pattern was also observed in illiterate adults (Ardila & Rosselli, 1989). Usually, older children, as well as literate adults, copy the design from left to right.

The effects of age, sex, and education (Ardila, Rosselli, & Rosas, 1989; Rosselli & Ardila, 1991) have been demonstrated in the copying of the Rey-Osterrieth Complex Figure. The score for normal adults in the immediate recall of the Rey-Osterrieth Complex Figure is 22 (Lezak, 1983). Normally, subjects retain about 60% of the figure. There are no normative values for delayed recall, but studies using the Taylor figures suggest that there is little loss after 1 hour in normal subjects (Mesulam, 1985). There are no norms for the copy or recall of the Rey-Osterrieth Complex Figure for subjects older than 60 years.

Normative Data

We completed two normative studies. In the first study, the influence of literacy was analyzed: the Rey-Osterrieth Complex Figure was given to subjects belonging to two extreme educational groups (totally illiterate and professional), with 100 subjects in each group. Subjects were divided by sex and age, with five age ranges (16–25, 26–35, 36–45, 46–55, and 56–65 years). Copying of the Rey-Osterrieth Complex Figure was scored following Taylor's system. Table 4.1 shows the obtained results. Professionals performed significantly better than illiterates, with this difference being more evident in the older group. There was an interaction of age and sex with educational level: in the professional group no differences were found between the male and female group, nor among the different age groups. In the illiterate group, however, males performed significantly

TABLE 4.1. Scores on Copying the Rey-Osterrieth Complex Figure for Normal Subjects Grouped by Age, Sex, and Two Extreme Educational Levels (N = 200)

Education	Age				
	16–25	26–35	36–45	46–55	56–65
Illiterates					
Male	21.7	25.2	25.3	22.6	12.0
Female	19.7	16.7	13.1	14.5	10.6
Professionals					
Male	35.5	35.6	34.3	34.9	34.7
Female	35.1	35.3	34.1	35.2	34.8

better than females, with a clear effect of age—the younger groups performed better than the oldest group.

Our second normative study analyzed the influence of age on the Rey-Osterrieth Complex Figure Test. Table 4.2 shows the results obtained in 346 subjects older than 55 years. Subjects were grouped according to age (five ranges), educational level (three levels), and sex, with 11 or 12 subjects in each cell. Scores negatively correlated with

TABLE 4.2. Scores on Copying the Rey-Osterrieth Complex Figure for Normal Subjects Grouped by Age, Sex, and Educational Level (N = 346)

Education (years)	Age (years)				
	55–59	60–65	66–70	71–75	>75
0–5					
Male	26.71	23.55	23.95	17.44	17.80
Female	24.60	20.00	15.60	13.77	10.33
6–12					
Male	32.67	28.64	26.50	22.86	16.09
Female	30.38	26.03	22.23	20.59	18.75
>12					
Male	31.42	30.91	30.50	26.64	21.79
Female	32.25	31.98	30.36	24.68	19.36
Mean	29.67	26.85	24.86	20.99	17.34

age, with a decrease particularly evident after 70 years. Men outperformed women in the lower educational group.

Table 4.3 presents immediate recall scores of the aforementioned subjects for the Rey-Osterrieth Complex Figure Test. There is a decrease of about 60% in the immediate recall score for patients. However, the loss between the copy and the immediate recall is higher in the older groups.

Norms (percentages, percentiles, and T scores) were obtained for the following four educational and age groups: age 55–65 years and 0–5 years of formal education; age 55–65 years and more than 5 years of formal education; over age 65 years and 0–5 years of formal education; and over age 65 years and more than 5 years of formal education (see Appendix B, Table B8).

Results in Brain-Damaged Populations

Patients with right-hemisphere damage tend to do more poorly than those with left-hemisphere damage on the Rey-Osterrieth Complex Figure (Lezak, 1983), with both groups presenting a significant number of errors (Binder, 1982). Hemineglect and asymmetric performance are characteristic of right-hemisphere–damaged patients. Asymmetry in copying is not so common in cases of left-hemisphere

TABLE 4.3. Scores on Copying the Rey-Osterrieth Complex Figure Test for Normal Subjects Grouped by Age, Educational Level, and Sex (N = 346)

Education (years)	Age (years)				
	55–59	60–65	66–70	71–75	>75
0–5					
Male	12.25	10.41	6.45	6.67	4.10
Female	10.00	6.91	4.35	3.59	3.00
6–12					
Male	17.58	12.23	11.89	10.36	4.95
Female	10.13	10.33	7.35	4.36	3.96
>12					
Male	17.92	15.82	13.23	10.91	8.75
Female	12.25	13.09	12.14	10.36	5.73
Mean	12.99	11.99	9.62	7.74	5.10

damage, although it can be present. Right-hemisphere–damaged patients usually produce a copy with superior integration and organization of the parts on the right side of the figure; conversely, left-hemisphere–damaged patients produce copies superior in quality and quantity of detail for the left side.

Poor performance on this test has been found in patients with focal damage in different locations, particularly in the right-parietal area (Lezak, 1983; Messerli, Seron, & Tissot, 1979; Pillon, 1981). In cases of left-hemisphere damage, delayed recall performance on the Rey-Osterrieth Complex Figure Test may be impaired, with an absence of the internal details of the figure. This is especially the case with left-frontotemporal damage (Kaplan, 1988). In patients with Alzheimer's disease, severe difficulties in recall of the figure can be considered an early clinical sign.

DRAW-A-CUBE TEST

Background

Constructional apraxia refers to a deficit in combining or organizing activity, a perceptuomotor activity, in which details must be clearly perceived and in which the relationships among the component parts of the entity must be apprehended if the desired synthesis of or composite of these parts is to be achieved (Benton, 1967). Kleist introduced in 1912 the term "optic apraxia" to describe the difficulties that patients with brain damage frequently have in performing visually guided movements. In 1912, Kleist proposed using "constructional apraxia" to describe disturbances in formative activities (like drawing and assembling cubes) in which the visuospatial arrangement of an object is lost but there is no apraxia for single movements. Some authors have preferred to use the name "apractoagnosia" (Lange, 1936; Luria, 1966) to emphasize the fact that this is an intermediate syndrome between apraxia and agnosia since it is neither a purely apraxic disorder nor a purely agnostic one. Only when a motor activity is under visuoperceptual control will the defect be apparent.

Constructional apraxia has been tested for with a variety of activities: drawing, arranging sticks in simple geometrical shapes, assembling blocks in a three-dimensional pattern, and arranging multicolored blocks into patterns of increasing complexity (Gainotti,

1985). Drawing is perhaps the most frequently used test, given its simplicity. Subjects are instructed to draw from memory or by copying, a drawing of a square, a cross, a cube, a house, a bicycle, or a complex nonsense figure may be requested. Only pencil and paper are required, and it is easy to test the patient at the bedside.

A quick and easy test of constructional ability is the Draw-a-Cube Test. Many clinical neuropsychologists include this test as a general screening device, particularly in patients with right-hemisphere damage. The ease and speed of administration of the Draw-a-Cube test are important advantages. Two different procedures of administration are used in neuropsychological practice: the subject is instructed to draw the cube from memory ("Please try to draw a cube as best you can") or to copy the cube from a drawing. Constructional difficulties are evident under both conditions.

Norms for the general population are not available. In children, a correlation has been observed between performance in cube drawing and age (e.g., Freeman, 1986, 1987), with young children experiencing difficulties representing three dimensions in their drawing; after around 12 years of age, children's drawings are similar to adults.

The Draw-a-Cube Test is extremely sensitive to educational and cultural variables (e.g., Ardila, Rosselli, & Rosas, 1989; Deregowski, 1986). Recognizing schematized figures is a highly trained ability that is often taken for granted. People without training in this ability cannot copy diagrams without introducing spatial distortion, such as rotating angles (Deregowski, 1986), and are unable to reproduce complex geometric patterns. For example, the difficulties found in children are similar to those observed in illiterates.

Normative Data

The Draw-a-Cube Test was given to subjects belonging to two extreme educational groups (illiterates and professionals), with 100 subjects in each group. Both male and females subjects were divided into five age ranges (16–25, 26–35, 36–45, 46–55, and 56–65 years). A drawing of a cube in black ink on white paper was presented to the subject with the instruction to copy the figure (see Appendix A15 for a reproduction of the figure used). No time limit was used. After the subject had finished the copy, the test figure was withdrawn and the subject was asked to draw the figure again (immediate recall); 20 minutes later the subject was asked to draw the figure once more (delayed recall).

The scoring system was based on seven components, each of which was scored 2 if correctly located and 1 if incorrectly located (maximum score = 14).

Table 4.4 presents the scores obtained by subjects of two different educational level groups. Professionals performed virtually perfectly under the three conditions; indeed, the differences between performance in the copying and recall situations were nonsignificant for this group. In the recall situations these subjects were probably not using a recently stored memory of the figure; instead, they were drawing the standard cube they had learned to draw previously, tapping into long-term memory. By contrast, illiterates presented a significant decrement in their scores across age groups and between experimental situations (copy, immediate recall, delayed recall); males did significantly better than females.

Results in Brain-Damaged Patients

Since the initial observations of constructional disorders, it has been emphasized that drawing difficulties are typically observed in cases of right-hemisphere damage (e.g., Lange, 1936). Further research confirmed the difficulties of right-hemisphere–damaged patients in

TABLE 4.4.   Scores Obtained by Normal Subjects on
the Draw-a-Cube Test (Copy, Immediate Recall, and Delayed Recall)
by Age, Educational Level and Sex (N = 200)

Educational level and age (years)	Copy		Immediate recall		Delayed recall	
	Males	Females	Males	Females	Males	Females
Illiterates						
16–25	9.1	4.5	7.3	4.5	6.5	4.2
26–35	8.7	3.3	6.5	3.3	5.3	3.0
36–45	6.5	3.4	5.8	3.3	5.1	2.9
46–55	5.0	3.5	3.8	2.9	3.1	2.6
56–65	3.5	3.5	3.7	3.1	3.1	2.5
Professionals						
16–25	13.9	13.7	13.6	13.6	13.7	13.7
26–35	13.8	13.9	13.7	13.5	13.7	13.9
36–45	13.7	13.7	13.6	13.4	13.6	13.4
46–55	13.9	13.9	13.5	13.7	13.9	13.9
56–65	13.6	13.6	13.1	13.7	13.3	13.7

drawing (Hecaen et al., 1961; McFie & Zangwill, 1960). Consequently, constructional apraxia syndrome was related to right-hemisphere dysfunction. However, drawing difficulties are also observed in cases of left-hemisphere damage (Piercy, Hecaen, & Ajuriaguerra, 1960), although the specific deficits in drawing are different (see Table 4.5). Most severe constructional deficits are observed in cases of parietal and right occipitoparietal damage, although patients with right frontal damage also present spatial difficulties in copying figures or drawing from memory.

It is worth noting that the ability to use three-dimensionality in drawing, and to draw in general, is especially sensitive to aging (Ardila & Rosselli, 1989). Difficulties in drawing are even observed during the fifth decade of life and correlate with the general decrease in performance abilities. However, drawing difficulties are observed especially in patients with dementia, and the diagnosis of Alzheimer's disease usually correlates with difficulties in drawing (Rosen, 1983). Since constructional apraxia usually is an early clinical sign in Alzheimer's disease (Ardila & Rosselli, 1986, 1992), constructional testing is critical in assessing dementia.

In cases of corpus callosum commissurotomy, it has been observed that the patient is more successful drawing a three-dimensional cube with his or her left, rather than right, hand. Perspective is observed and adequate spatial relations between lines are evident, although the motor act is clumsy owing to the lack of skill and training in drawing with the non-dominant hand. When such patients attempt the Draw-a-Cube Test with the dominant hand, the drawing lacks the three-dimensional quality and is spatially inade-

TABLE 4.5.   Characteristics of Drawings by Patients
with Right- and Left-Hemisphere Damage

Right-hemisphere damage	Left-hemisphere damage
Better on right	Better on left
Drawn from right to left	Drawn from left to right
Microreproduction	Macroreproduction
Absence of configuration	Absence of internal details
More elements than in model	Fewer elements than in model
Incorrectly oriented in space	Correctly oriented in space
Iteration of lines	Simplification of lines
Fragmented and scattered	Coherent but simplified

quate (Bogen, 1985); that is, there is a sort of constructional apraxia observed with the dominant hand performance.

Summary

In summary, the following points can be made:

1. For the well-educated subjects in our study, performance on the Draw-a-Cube Test was virtually perfect. No effect of age or sex was found for the copy, immediate recall, or delayed recall conditions of the test.

2. For illiterate subjects, scores were only about 35% of the score earned by professional individuals. It was virtually impossible for the former to indicate three dimensions in the cube drawing. Significant age and sex effects were observed: Males outperformed females, with the latter obtaining about 60% of the male copy score. With each successive age range studied, a decrease in score of about 15% was observed. There was a decrease in performance between the copy and the immediate recall condition, and between the latter and the delayed recall condition.

3. Owing to its high sensitivity to educational factors, it is not advisable to use the Draw-a-Cube Test with low-education level subjects (either by instructing them to copy a drawing of a cube or by having them reproduce one from memory). In high-education level subjects, this can be a test very sensitive to brain dysfunction even with populations after the seventh decade of life.

FINGER-TAPPING TEST

Background

The Finger-Tapping Test is one of the most commonly used tests of manual agility and has been a part of the Halstead-Reitan Neuropsychological Battery. It consists of a tapping key attached to a counter (Halstead, 1947). Five consecutive 10-second trials are allotted for each hand, with the hand held in a constant position in order to make the required movements of only one finger. The score of each hand is the average after five trials. According to Reitan and Wolfson (1985), normal individuals show an average of 50 taps for the right hand and 45 taps for the left hand per 10-second period. There are some significant differences according to sex, with better performance in males. When using the preferred hand, males earn a mean score of around 56±5, females 51±5 (Dodrill, 1979). There is a tendency for the score to decrease with age appearing at around 50–60 years (Harley, Levthold, Matthews, & Bergs, 1980).

It has been observed that concurrent performance of some other activity interferes with tapping performance, particularly simultaneous verbal activity, which decreases the performance with the right hand but not with the left (e.g., Ikeda, 1987). Results using other cognitive tasks have not yielded clear results (Dalen & Hugdahl, 1988).

Bornstein (1986) has criticized the current cutoff scores used in the tapping test, emphasizing the necessity of adjusting conventional cutoff scores for subject variables.

Normative Data

The Finger-Tapping Test was administered to 348 subjects divided into groups according to age (56–60, 61–65, 66–70, 71–75, and more than 75 years), sex, and educational level (0–5, 6–12, and more than 12 years of formal education). The influence of sex was statistically significant: males (the mean for performance with the preferred hand was 41.19, for the nonpreferred hand 38.29) had a better performance than females (the mean for the preferred hand was 35.12, for the nonpreferred hand 32.99). Table 4.6 presents the results obtained in different age and educational groups.

Norms (percentages, percentiles, and T scores) were obtained for the following four educational and age groups: age 55–65 years and

TABLE 4.6. Means of Scores Earned by Normal
Subjects on the Finger-Tapping Test
According to Age and Education
(Nonpreferred Hand Scores in Parentheses)

Education (years)	Age (years)				
	56–60	61–65	66–70	71–75	>75
0–5	40.89	39.71	32.68	32.37	26.15
	(37.21)	(36.24)	(31.63)	(29.68)	(26.60)
6–12	44.42	43.25	39.83	36.20	30.00
	(39.92)	(39.21)	(37.04)	(35.23)	(27.65)
>12	48.08	41.67	40.04	39.40	33.52
	(46.29)	(39.57)	(37.54)	(35.95)	(31.29)

0–5 years of formal education; age 55–65 years and more than 5 years of formal education; over age 65 years and 0–5 years of formal education; and over age 65 years and more than 5 years of formal education (see Appendix B, Table 9).

Results in Brain-Damaged Populations

Scores on the Finger-Tapping Test decrease after brain damage in general. Unilateral lesions result in slowing in performance by the contralateral hand (Finlayson & Reitan, 1980). This appears to be particularly true in the case of anterior lesions and is less significant after posterior cerebral damage.

Pruebas Neuropsicologicas para Hispanoparlantes

A1. Versión Española del Examen Breve del Estado Mental

Nombre _____   Edad _____

Escolaridad _____   Fecha _____

Examinador _____

ORIENTACION

Puntaje

En qué año estamos?	0	1
En qué fecha estamos?	0	1
Qué horas son aproximadamente?*	0	1
Qué dia de a semana es hoy?	0	1
En qué mes estamos?	0	1
En qué provincia (departamento, estado) estamos?	0	1
En qué pais estamos?	0	1
En qué ciudad estamos?	0	1
En qué sitio estamos?	0	1
En qué piso estamos?	0	1

RETENCION

"Repita despues de mi las siguientes palabras": TORMENTA, LEON, ZAPATO   0   1   2   3

(Un segundo de intervalo entre las palabras y un punto por cada palabra correcta.) Luego, repítalas hasta que el sujeto logre decir las tres palabras. Anote el número de ensayos utilizados. _____

ATENCION Y CALCULO   0   1   2   3   4   5

Serie del 7 (100-7) ("Reste sucesivamente 7 a partir de 100.") Suspenda la prueba luego de cinco respuestas. Dé un punto por cada respuesta correcta.

---

*Se acepta una hora de error como normal.

From Folstein, M. F., Folstein, S. E., & McHugh, P. A. (1975). *Journal of Psychiatric Research*, 13 189–198. Reprinted by permission of the authors.

EVOCACION   0   1   2   3

Pidale al sujeto que recuerde las tres palabras presentadas anterior-
mente. De 1 punto por cada palabra correctamente evocada

LENGUAJE

Denomine: LAPIZ, RELOJ   0   1   2
Repita: "NI SIS, NI NOS NI PEROS"   0   1
Ejecute la siguiente orden: "TOME ESTE PAPEL   0   1   2   3
CON SU MANO DERECHA, DOBLELO POR LA
MITAD Y COLOQUELO EN EL PISO"
Lea y siga la siguiente instruccion: CIERRE LOS   0   1
OJOS
Escriba una frase cualquiera   0   1

COPIA   0   1

"Copie el siguiente diseno"

                                    Puntaje Total   _____

Figura para el examen del estado mental:

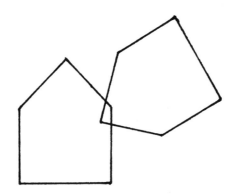

A2. Prueba de Cancelación

```
B  S  A  P  G  Q  T  V  E  X  A  C  B  Y  W  P  K  N  A  F
O  T  M  C  L  N  D  U  V  C  H  M  G  T  R  A  B  D  V  X
Z  L  S  Y  W  A  N  N  T  E  G  A  K  O  A  V  S  J  C  E
W  D  Q  Z  B  H  R  Z  D  U  S  Y  A  L  I  Z  A  B  D  P
A  N  C  U  F  G  R  A  F  J  Q  H  R  F  M  G  W  F  T  C
Q  W  N  P  L  C  I  T  V  K  U  E  Z  L  C  H  S  H  I  O
V  A  X  R  B  J  C  A  W  E  S  C  U  F  I  A  R  Z  A  I
G  O  U  A  N  G  U  Z  H  W  D  T  Q  C  J  N  V  W  K  E
```

Tiempo ———

Correctas (16) ———

Omisiones ———

Adiciones ———

A3. Prueba de Denominación para Hispanoparlantes

Nombre _____   Edad _____

Escolaridad _____   Fecha _____

Examinador _____

Latencia de la respuesta	Figura	Correcta sin clave	Clave semántica	Clave fonológica
_____	ARBOL (una planta)	_____	_____	_____
_____	TIJERAS (para cortar)	_____	_____	_____
_____	LLAVE (para abrir)	_____	_____	_____
_____	RELOJ (para la hora)	_____	_____	_____
_____	CORBATA (de vestir)	_____	_____	_____
_____	GUITARRA (un instrumento musical)	_____	_____	_____
_____	BISAGRA (de la puerta)	_____	_____	_____
_____	EMBUDO (para verter líquidos)	_____	_____	_____
_____	TERMOMETRO (mide la temperatura)	_____	_____	_____
_____	CAMELLO (un animal)	_____	_____	_____
_____	JIRAFA (un animal)	_____	_____	_____
_____	ALICANTES (herramienta)	_____	_____	_____
_____	BANDERA (símbolo del país)	_____	_____	_____
_____	CASCO (del minero)	_____	_____	_____
_____	RASTRILLO (de agricultura)	_____	_____	_____

1. Número de Respuestas Correctas   = _____ × 3 = _____
   Espontáneamente

2. Número de Respuestas Correctas con   = _____ × 2 = _____
   Clave Semántica

3. Número de Respuestas con Clave   = _____ × 1 = _____
   Fonológica

Puntaje Total = _____

A4. Prueba de Lectura para Hispanoparlantes
(Utilice las láminas L-1, L-2, L-3, L-4,
L-5, L-6, L-7, L-8, y L-9)

Nombre _____   Edad _____

Escolaridad _____   Fecha _____

Examinador _____

---

1. *Lectura de letras* (Lámina L-1). Transcriba textualmente la respuesta del paciente. Si el paciente no puede leer o comete errores, póngalo a reconocer las mismas letras; utilice para el reconocimiento un orden diferente.

	Lectura	*Reconocimiento*
S		
E		
I		
O		
B		
n		
P		
m		
h		
A		
F		
T		
K		
L		
U		
N		
P		

Puntaje. _____ (Se califica el numero de errores en lectura. Puntaje máximo = 17.)

2. *Lectura de sílabas* (Lámina L-2). Transcriba textualmente la respuesta del paciente. Si el paciente no puede leer o comete errores, póngalo a reconocer las mismas sílabas; utilice para el reconocimiento un orden diferente.

Lectura	*Reconocimiento*
PA	
TE	
LI	
TUS	
PIL	
CLUS	
TRANS	
ta	
pi	
cla	
bra	
tla	

Puntaje. _____ (Cada sílaba se califica "0" si es leída correctamente, y "1" si hay errores. Puntaje maximo = 12.)

3. *Lectura de logotomas* (Lámina L-3). Transcriba textualmente la respuesta del paciente. Si el paciente no puede leer o comete errores, pongalo a reconocer los mismo logotomas; utilice para el reconocimiento un orden diferente.

Lectura	*Reconocimiento*
talo	
pigla	

Lectura	Reconocimiento

estigo

orgo

asrilo

artaglo

rada

jara

tacama

fasaja

badiga

Puntaje. _____ (Cada logotoma se califica "0" si es leído correctamente, y "1" si hay errores. Puntaje máximo = 11.)

4. *Lectura de palabras* (Lámina L-4). Transcriba textualmente la respuesta del paciente. Si el paciente no puede leer o comete errores, póngalo a reconocer las mismas palabras; utilice para el reconocimiento un orden diferente.

Lectura	Reconocimiento

casa

libro

huevo

ventana

caballo

bicicleta

dromedario

dactilografía

despilfarrar

glacilidad

Lectura   Reconocimiento

arremolinar

prepotencia

Puntaje. ____ (Cada palabra se califica "0" si es leída correctamente, y "1" si hay errores. Puntaje maximo = 12.)

NOTA: El reconocimiento se utiliza para un análisis cualitativo.

5. *Lectura de frases* (Lámina L-5). Transcriba textualmente la respuesta del paciente.

La cantina es de Juan _____.

Miguel necesita zapatos _____.

La gente se reune en la plaza _____.

El niño tiró la caja de galletas al río _____.

Algunos gusanos se transforman en mariposas _____.

Puntaje. ____ (Cada frase se califica "0" si es leída correctamente, y "1" si hay errores. Puntaje máximo = 12

6. *Comprensión de órdenes escritas* (Lámina L-6). Pida al paciente que lea mentalmente las siguientes órdenes y las ejecute.

Correcto   Incorrecto

Cierre los ojos

Tóquese la oreja

Con su mano derecha muéstreme su boca

Levante su mano pero no se toque la nariz

No me dé el lápiz sino las llaves

Dése un beso en la nariz

Levante un brazo y abra la boca

Mire el techo y despues el piso

Tóquese la oreja despues de tocarse la nariz

Puntaje. ——— (Cada orden se califica "0" si es realizada correctamente, y "1" si hay errores. Puntaje máximo = 9.)

OBSERVACIONES

7. *Lectura de un Texto* (Láminas L-7 y L-8). Pida al paciente que lea en voz alta el texto de la Lámina L-7. El examinador debe tomar el tiempo total y marcar únicamente los errores debajo de la palabra correspondiente

El gusano y la mariposa

Dos gusanos cayeron en el agua. Uno de ellos pensó que era inútil tratar de salvarse ya que nunca lograría llegar hasta la orilla. Se dejó entonces llevar por la corriente y se ahogó.
　　El otro trató de salir. Pensó que quizas lo lograría. Que era mejor intentar que dejarse llevar por la corriente y ahogarse inevitablemente. Entonces nado con todas sus fuerzas por un largo rato.
　　Cuando ya pensaba que no podría más y que aún la orilla estaba muy lejos, sintió que se convertía en mariposa y le aparecían unas enormes alas en su espalda. Entonces salió volandó y escapo de morir ahogado.

Tiempo ———

Puntaje ——— (número total de paralexias)

8. *Comprension de Lectura en Voz Alta.* Cuando el paciente termine de leer, presentele las preguntas de la lamina L-8.

　　　　　　1. A　B　C
　　　　　　2. A　B　C
　　　　　　3. A　B　C
　　　　　　4. A　B　C

Puntaje de Comprensión de Lectura en Voz Alta ——— (número total de errores. Puntaje máximo = 4.)

OBSERVACIONES

9. *Comprensión de lectura silenciosa* (Lámina L-9). Pídale al paciente que lea para sí mismo el texto de la lámina L-9. Cuando haya terminado, anote el tiempo y formúlele las siguientes preguntas:

1. Cuál es la idea central de la historia? _____
2. Cómo se encontraron los dos primitivos? _____
3. Cuál fue la reacción que tuvieron al verse? _____
4. Qué pasó en el momento en que iban a pelearse? _____
5. Qué es lo que nos enseña esta historia? _____

Tiempo _____

Puntaje de Comprensión de Lectura Silenciosa _____ (Califique "0" si las respuestas corresponden al contenido de la historia, y "1" si no corresponden o el paciente muestra no recordar. Puntaje máximo = 5.)

OBSERVACIONES

Resumen de los Puntajes

1. (Lectura de Letras + Lectura de Sílabas)/2 _____
2. Lectura de Logotomas _____
3. (Lectura de Palabras + Lectura de Frases)/2 _____
4. Comprensión de Ordenes Escritas _____
5. Numero de Paralexias en un Texto _____
6. (Comprensión de Lectura en Voz Alta + Comprensión de Lectura Silenciosa)/2 _____

Puntaje Total de Errores _____

Corrección por Escolaridad _____

Puntaje Final Corregido _____
Corrección por escolaridad para la prueba de lectura.

Años de Educación	Corrección
<5 años	−6
6–12 años	−3
>12 años	−0

Láminas L-1, L-2, L-3, L-4, L-5, L-6, L-7, L-8, L-9

SEIO

BnPmh

AFTKLUNP

L-1

PA TE LI TUS PIL CLUS TRANS

ta pi cla bra tla

L-2

talo pigla estigo orgo asrilo

artaglo rada jara tacama fasaja

badiga

L-3

CASA LIBRO VENTANA

CABALLO BICICLETA HUEVO

DROMEDARIO DACTILOGRAFIA

DESPILFARRAR GLACILIDAD

ARREMOLINAR PREPOTENCIA

L-4

La cantina es de Juan

Miguel necesita zapatos

La gente se reune en la plaza

El niño tiró la caja de galletas al río

Algunos gusanos se transforman en mariposas

L-5

Cierre los ojos

Tóquese la oreja

Con su mano derecha muéstreme su boca

Levante su mano pero no se toque la nariz

No me dé el lápiz sino las llaves

Dese un beso en la nariz

Levante un brazo y abra la boca

Mire el techo y después el piso

Tóquese la oreja antes de tocarse la nariz

L-6

EL GUSANO Y LA MARIPOSA

DOS GUSANOS CAYERON EN EL AGUA.

UNO DE ELLOS PENSÓ QUE ERA INÚTIL TRATAR DE SALVARSE YA QUE NUNCA LOGRARIA LLEGAR HASTA LA ORILLA. SE DEJO ENTONCES LLEVAR POR LA CORRIENTE Y SE AHOGÓ.

EL OTRO TRATÓ DE SALIR. PENSÓ QUE QUIZÁS LO LOGRARÍA. QUE ERA MEJOR INTENTAR QUE DEJARSE LLEVAR POR LA CORRIENTE Y AHOGARSE INEVITABLEMENTE. ENTONCES NADÓ CON TODAS SUS FUERZAS POR UN LARGO RATO.

CUANDO YA PENSABA QUE NO PODÍA MÁS Y QUE AÚN LA ORILLA ESTABA MUY LEJOS, SINTIÓ QUE SE CONVERTÍA EN MARIPOSA Y LE APARECIÁN UNAS ENORMES ALAS EN SU ESPALDA. ENTONCES SALIÓ VOLANDO Y ESCAPÓ DE MORIR AHOGADO.

L-7

1. CUÁNTOS GUSANOS CAYERON AL AGUA
   - A. UNO
   - B. DOS
   - C. TRES

2. POR QUÉ SE AHOGÓ EL PRIMER GUSANO
   - PORQUE NO SABÍA NADAR
   - PORQUE PENSÓ QUE SERÍA INÚTIL LUCHAR
   - PORQUE ERA MÁS DEBIL

3. QUÉ PASÓ CON EL SEGUNDO GUSANO
   - TAMBIÉN SE AHOGÓ
   - CREYÓ QUE SE AHOGARÍA
   - TRATÓ DE SALIR

4. CÓMO SE SALVÓ EL OTRO GUSANO
   - PORQUE SE CONVIRTÍO EN MARIPOSA
   - PORQUE PUDO NADAR
   - PORQUE LO AYUDÓ UNA MARIPOSA

L-8

COMO NACIO LA SOCIEDAD HUMANA

Al llegar a la gruta que le servía de habitación, el hombre primitivo se detuvo asombrado y molesto. Qué occurría?

Otro hombre, establa sentado, junto a la boca de su caverna y parecia decir: "He aquí un buen lugar para guarecerme del frío y de la lluvia."

El primer hombre contrajo jos músculos, y avanzo amenazadoramente hacia el invasor. El intruso, a su vez, se puso de pié.

—   Deja esta caverna; me pertenece—decia la mirada cargada de odio,—del antiguo morador de la gruta.

—   Jamas—respondió, rabioso el otro. Ya iban a embestirse, cuando un formidable rugido los inmovilizó. Una enorme bestia trepaba por la ladera, era necesario intentar, rapidamente una defensa.

Los hombres se combrendieron con una mirada y uniendo sus fuerzas lograron impulsar un gran peñasco abajo, en dirección del animal. La roca, que un solo hombre no hubiera pudido empujar, alcanzó a la fiera antes de que pudiera ponerse a salvo.

Los dos hombres volvieron a mirarse. El odio había desaparecido de sus ojos. Entendieron que lo más conveniente era, en adelante, suma fuerzas.

Desde ese dia la caverna tuvo dos habitantes.

L-9

A5. Prueba de Escritura para Hispanoparlantes
(Utilice las láminas L-1, L-2, L-3, L-4 y L-5)

Nombre —————————————— Edad ————————————

Escolaridad —————————— Fecha ———————————

Examinador ——————————————

1. *Escritura de letras* (Lámina L-1). Dicte al paciente las letras que se encuentran en la lámina. Posteriormente, pídale que las copie. Utilice para ello una hoja en blanco.

Puntaje ——— (Se califica el número de errores. Cada letra se califica "0" si es escrita correctamente y "1" si hay errores. Puntaje máximo = 17.)

2. *Escritura de sílabas* (Lámina L-2). Dicte al paciente las silabas de la lamina L-2. Posteriormente, pídale que las copie.

Puntaje ——— (Cada sílaba se califica "0" si es escrita correctamente al dictado y 1 si hay errores. Puntaje máximo = 12.)

3. *Escritura de palabras* (Lámina L-4). Dicte al paciente las palabras de la lámina L-4. Posteriormente, pídale que las copie.

Puntaje ——— (Cada palabra se califica "0" si es escrita correctamente al dictado y 1 si hay errores. Puntaje maximo = 12.)

4. *Escritura de frases* (L-5). Dicte al paciente las frases de la lámina L-5. Posteriormente, pídale que las copie.

Puntaje ——— (Cada frase se califica "0" si es escrita correctamente al dictado y 1 si hay errores. Puntaje máximo = 5.)

NOTA: La copia no se califica y se utiliza unicamente para el análisis cualitativo.

5.1. *Transcripcion de letra cursiva a letra imprenta.* Pídale al paciente que transcriba las siguiente frases a letra de molde:

El nino camina por la calle

Puntaje _____ (Califique como "0" si el paciente logra cambiar el tipo de letra sin errores. "1" implica la presencia de errores en el cambio de letra)

5.2. *Transcripción de letra imprenta letra cursiva.* Pídale al paciente que transcriba a letra cursiva la siguiente frase

el hombre toma café

Puntaje _____ (Califique como "0" si el paciente logra cambiar el tipo de letra sin errores. "1" implica la presencia de errores en el cambio de letra)

5.3. *Transcripción de mayúsculas a minúsculas.* Pídale al paciente que cambie a minúscula la siguiente frase

EL CARRO AVANZA RAPIDAMENTE

Puntaje _____ (Califique como "0" si el paciente logra cambiar el tipo de letra sin errores. "1" implica la presencia de errores en el cambio de letra)

5.4. *Transcripción de minúsculas a mayúsculas.* Pídale al paciente que cambie a mayuscúlas la siguiente frase:

las naranjas crecen en los árboles.

Puntaje _____ (Califique como "0" si el paciente logra cambiar el tipo de letra sin errores. "1" implica la presencia de errores en el cambio de letra)

Puntaje total transcripciones (5.1 + 5.2 + 5.3 + 5.4) _____ (Puntaje máximo = 4)

6. *Descripción escrita de una lámina.* Pídale al paciente que en una hoja en blanco describa todo lo que esta sucediendo en una lámina. Utilice por ejemplo la Lamina 1 de la Prueba de Boston para el Diagnóstico de las Afasias (Goodglass & Kaplan, 1972, 1979, 1983).

Puntaje _____ Califique como "0" si el paciente logra una escritura normal. 1 si por lo menos hay dos ideas escritas adecuadamente. 2 si por lo menos hay una frase escrita adecuadamente, pero sin secuencia de ideas. 3 si hay por lo menos entre una y cuatro palabras reconocibles y relacionadas con el dibujo. 4 si la escritura es ilegible; no hay sustantivos o verbos reconocibles.

OBSERVACIONES

Rusumen de los Puntajes

1. (Escritura de letras, sílabas, palabras y frases)/4 _____
2. Transcripciones _____
3. Descripción escrita de una lámina _____
   Puntaje Total de Errores _____
   Corrección por Escolaridad _____
   Puntaje Final Corregido _____

Corrección por escolaridad para la prueba de escritura:

Años de Educación	*Escolaridad*
<5 anos	−3
6–12 anos	−1
>12 anos	0

A6. Prueba de Repetición para Hispanoparlantes

Nombre —————————————— Edad ————————————

Escolaridad —————————————— Fecha ————————————

Examinador ——————————————

I. *Repetición de fonemas*

A   I   E   O   U

TA PA BA DA KA GA JA MA CHA NA NA
RA SA RA LA YA FA SA

Puntaje ——— (Califique "0" si el fonema es correctamente repetido; 1 si hay algún error. Puntaje máximo = 23.)

II. *Repetición de sílabas*

TLA TRA CLA CRA BRA BLA PLAN CONS TRANS

Puntaje ——— (Califique "0" si la silaba es correctamente repetida; 1 si hay algún error. Puntaje máximo = 9.)

III. *Repetición de logotomas*

PAFA BAFA PAMA LADA NALA RALA LARRA
RARA RADA TARA TASA TADA TANA CATA TAGA
TAJA PATACA TAPAGA BADAGA GABADA MANANA
NAMANA FASAJA SAFAJA

Puntaje ——— (Califique "0" si el logotoma correctamente repetido; 1 si hay algún error. Puntaje máximo = 24.)

IV. *Pares mínimos*

PALA–BALA FUENTE–PUENTE MATA–BATA MOTO–MOZO
CODO–CONO HORA–OLA CERRO–CERO HOYO–OCHO
CANA–CALLA CARRO–JARRO HIGO–HIJO PISO–PESO
PALO–PELO LONA–LUNA

Puntaje ——— (Califique "0" si el par es correctamente repetido; 1 si hay algún error. Puntaje máximo = 14.)

V. Repetición de palabras

1. PAN
2. SOL
3. CASA
4. MESA
5. LIBRO
6. BRAZO
7. CABALLO
8. VENTANA
9. BICICLETA
10. DROMEDARIO
11. PLANETARIO
12. CONSIDERACION
13. DESENMASCARAR
14. DACTILOGRAFIA
15. PRESTIDIGITACION

Puntaje _____ (Califique "0" si la palabra es correctamente repetida; 1 si hay algún error. Puntaje máximo = 15.)

VI. Repeticion de frases

1. El niño llora. (3)*
2. Los limones son ácidos. (4)
3. Pedro camina por la calle. (5)
4. Las naranjas crecen en los árboles. (6)
5. La escuela tiene cinco salones de clase. (7)
6. Ayer en la tarde cayó un fuerte aguacero. (8)
7. Por la mañana la radio anunció las nuevas noticias (9)
8. El carro verde avanza por la nueva autopista a gran velocidad. (10)
9. El presidente de la republica fue elegido esta mañana por el pueblo (12)
10. La niña sale para la escuela con el libro que compró su mamá. (13)
11. El acrobata del circo se presentará en la función del sabado por la tarde. (14)

*En paréntesis el número de palabras in cada frase.

12. Los elefantes son animales que se alimentan de las hojas que crecen en los árboles. (15)

13. A pesar de las dificultades que tuvo durante el año, el estudiante logró pasar todos los exámenes (17)

14. Todos los implementos que se necesitan para estudiar en la universidad, los venden en la tienda de la esquina. (19)

15. Los medio modernos de comunicación constituyen un sistema para acortar las distancias entre los hombres que viven en diferentes países. (20).

Puntaje _____ (Califique "0" si la frase es correctamente repetida; 1 si hay algún error. Puntaje máximo = 15)

Resumen de los Puntajes

1. Repetición de fonemas   ——

2. Repetición de silabas   ——

3. Repetición de logotomas   ——

4. Repetición de pares mínimos   ——

5. Repetición de palabras   ——

6. Repetición de frases   ——

Puntaje Total de Errores   ——

Corrección por Escolaridad   ——

Puntaje Final Corregido   ——

Corrección por escolaridad para la prueba de repetición

Años de Educación	Corrección
<6 años	−13
6–12 años	−9
>12 años	−4

A7. Prueba de Discriminación Fonológica
para Hispanoparlantes

Nombre _____   Edad _____

Escolaridad _____   Fecha _____

Examinador _____

Son iguales (I) o diferentes (D)?

		Diferentes	Iguales
1.	PALA–BALA (D)	_____	_____
2.	PALA–PALA (I)	_____	_____
3.	BESO–BESO (I)	_____	_____
4.	PESO–BESO (D)	_____	_____
5.	HIGO–HIJO (D)	_____	_____
6.	HIJO–HIJO (I)	_____	_____
7.	GARRA–GARRA (I)	_____	_____
8.	JARRA–GARRA (D)	_____	_____
9.	TORO–TORO (I)	_____	_____
10.	CORO–CORO (I)	_____	_____
11.	TUNA–CUNA (D)	_____	_____
12.	CUNA–CUNA (I)	_____	_____
13.	FUENTE–PUENTE (D)	_____	_____
14.	FUENTE–FUENTE (I)	_____	_____
15.	FARRA–PARRA (D)	_____	_____
16.	FARRA–FARRA (I)	_____	_____
17.	OLA–HORA (D)	_____	_____
18.	HORA–OLA (D)	_____	_____
19.	PELO–PELO (I)	_____	_____
20.	PERO–PERO (I)	_____	_____
21.	MANO–MALO (D)	_____	_____
22.	MANO–MANO (I)	_____	_____

	Diferentes	Iguales
23. PALA–PALA (I)	——	——
24. PANA–PANA (I)	——	——
25. BATA–MATA (D)	——	——
26. MATA–BATA (D)	——	——
27. SUBA–SUMA (D)	——	——
28. SUBA–SUMA (D)	——	——
29. CORO–CORO (I)	——	——
30. CORRO–CORRO (I)	——	——
31. MORO–MORRO (D)	——	——
32. MORRO–MORO (D)	——	——
33. PALA–MALA (D)	——	——
34. MALA–MALA (I)	——	——
35. TIA–TIA (I)	——	——
36. DIA–TIA (D)	——	——
37. VIENTO–VIENTO (I)	——	——
38. VIENTO–VIENDO (D)	——	——
39. CACHO–CAYO (D)	——	——
40. CAYO–CAYO (I)	——	——

Respuestas correctas *iguales*	——	Respuestas incorrectas *iguales*	——
Respuestas correctas *diferentes*	——	Respuestas incorrectas *diferentes*	——
Total de respuestas correctas	——	Total de respuestas incorrectas	——
Porcentaje correcto	——		

A8. Prueba de Gramática para Hispanoparlantes

Nombre ———————————— Edad ——————————

Escolaridad ———————————— Fecha ——————————

Examinador ————————————

1. LENGUAJE ESPONTANEO (se sugiere utilizar una grabadora)
   Cuénteme todo lo que está sucediendo en esta lámina (Utilice por
   ejemplo la Lamina 1 de la Prueba de Boston para el Diagnóstico de
   las Afasias; Goodglass & Kaplan, 1972.)

_____

_____

_____

_____

_____

_____

_____

_____

_____

_____

1.1. Número de sustantivos ——; 1.2. número de verbos ——;
1.3. número de adjetivos;   1.4. conectores gramaticales ——;
1.5. número total de palabras ——

2. COMPLETAR LAS SEGUIENTES FRASES: VERBOS
   Coloque un verbo (o acción) correspondiente (v. gr., Esta mañana
   ——————— dos kilometros en el estadio. (El verbo correcto
   puede ser "corrí.")

   1. Ayer la secretaria ——————— una carta (escribió)*

   2. Juan tiene hambre; ahora el ——————— un pastel (se comera; se
      va a comer)

*Las respuestas correctas se encuentran en paréntesis.

3. La semana proxima Susana _____ una pelicula (ira a ver; vera)

4. Hubiera llegado temprano a tu casa si me _____ llamado antes (hubieras)

5. Suena el timbre, _____ la puerta (abre; ve a abrir)

Complete las frases siguientes colocando el verbo correspondiente en pasado (v. gr., Escribo una carta a mi mamá; ayer _____ una carta a mi mamá; la palabra correcta es "escribí").

6. Voy a decir su nombre; ayer _____ su nombre (dije)

7. Mi hermana coloca el libro sobre la mesa; hace una hora lo _____ sobre la mesa (colocó)

8. El esta jugando cartas; hace dos días el _____ cartas (jugó)

Pase a futuro las frases siguientes (v. gr., "ayer fuiste a cine; mañana _____ a cine." La palabra correcta es "irás.")

9. Hoy Mónica vino a saludarte; mañana ella _____ a saludarte (vendrá)

10. Ayer José fué a Panamá; la próxima semana José _____ a Panamá (irá)

11. Tú éstas trabajando en ventas; el próximo año _____ trabajando en ventas (estarás)

Complete las siguientes frases colocando el presente correspondiente (v. gr., "ayer estuve comiendo en un restaurante; ahora _____ comiendo en un restaurante"; la palabra correcta es "estoy").

12. Ayer escuché un concierto; ahora _____ un concierto (escucho, estoy escuchando)

13. Yo voy a ver una exposición. Ahora _____ una exposición (veo, estoy viendo)

14. Mi hijo estuvo enfermo. El ahora _____ enfermo (está)

Complete con el ver ir en su forma correspondiente las frases siguientes (v. gr., Todos los sábados _____ al cine con María; la forma correcta del verbo ir en este caso es "voy")

15. La semana pasada yo _____ a tu casa (fuí)

16. Ahora el niño _____ al parque (va)

17. Marta, Luis y tu _____ al centro de la ciudad esta tarde (iran, van a ir)

18. Hace un mes ellos _____ al museo (fueron)

19. Te prestaré el libro cuando _____ a mi casa (vengas)

Puntaje ____ (Número de errores. Puntaje máximo = 19)

3. COMPLETAR LAS SIGUIENTES FRASES: PREPOSICIONES
   Complete las siguientes frases utilizando la palabra más apropiada (v. gr., Roberto y Lucía fueron al parque _____ sus hijos. La forma más apropiada seria entonces "Roberto y Lucía fueron al parque con sus hijos")

1. María le regala _____ Andrés un libro interesante (a)

2. Los estudiantes van _____ la universidad (a, hacia)

3. Cuando me levanto por la mañana veo _____ Juanita pasar en bicicleta (a)

4. Los maestros de la escuela se asombraron _____ el buen rendimiento de los estudiantes (con, de)

5. _____ el gobierno pasado se realizaron muchos proyectos importantes (durante, en)

6. La mayoría de las personas escriben _____ la mano derecha (con)

7. Los niños salieron a pasear _____ sus padres (con)

8. Luisa colocó la mesa _____ la pared (contra)

9. Los militares ordenaron dispersar _____ enemigo (al)

10. Las señoras comieron _____ la casa de Elena (en)

11. La casa de Pedro se encuentra _____ las calles 2 y 3 (entre)

12. El carro _____ mi mamá es de color gris (de)

13. Siempre regreso _____ la oficina a las seis de la tarde (de)

14. Los periodistas hablaron _____ las proximas elecciones (sobre, de)

15. El almacén está abierto _____ las dos de la tarde hasta las cinco (desde)

16. Voy _____ el parque a trotar todos los días (a)

17. Sólo hay plazo para entregar los formularios _____ hoy (hasta)

18. Silvia compró un regalo _____ su mamá (para, a)

19. Mañana viajaremos _____ Santa Marta en el avión de la tarde (a)

20. Este juguete fué fabricado _____ Jaime (por)

21. El libro titulado "Cien Años de Soledad" fue escrito _____ García Márquez (por)

22. Mis amigos vinieron _____ mí, para llevarme al aeropuerto (por)

23. Los jóvenes que iban para México pasaron _____ Monterrey (por)

24. _____ como este el tiempo, el domingo iremos a la playa (según)

25. La señora salió a la calle _____ el paraguas y se mojó (sin)

26. Los libros estan _____ la mesa (sobre)

27. Los estudiantes hablaron _____ las enfermedades más comunes (de, sobre)

Puntaje ____. (Número de errores. Puntaje máximo = 27)

4. CONCORDANCIA: USO DE ARTICULOS
Señale el artículo correspondiente a las siguientes palabras (v. gr., si yo le digo "manos", usted me dice "las manos").

1. ____ casas (las)   7. ____ aguas (las)
2. ____ perro (el)   8. ____ azucar (el)
3. ____ telefonos (los)   9. ____ águila (el)
4. ____ lámpara (la)   10. ____ águilas (las)
5. ____ zapatos (los)   11. ____ arte (el)
6. ____ artes (las)   12. ____ agua (el)

Puntaje ____ (Número de errores. Puntaje máximo = 12.)

5. CONCORDANCIA: ADJETIVOS
Señale un adjetivo que sea aplicable a los siguientes sustantivos (v. gr., si yo le digo niña, usted me puede decir por ejemplo niña bonita, o niña inteligente).

1. libros _____   6. pensamientos _____
2. ciudad _____   7. opiniones _____
3. ciudadanos _____   8. casas _____
4. fila _____   9. aspecto _____
5. vidrio _____   10. caracter _____

Señale que puede ser o estar (v. gr., si yo le digo sucios, usted me señala cualquier cosa que pueda tener la caracteristica de estar sucia; por ejemplo, los zapatos)

11. interesante _____	16. bonitas _____
12. útiles _____	17. inquietos _____
13. enredadas _____	18. dudosas _____
14. simpáticas _____	19. feo _____
15. flacas _____	20. transparente _____

Puntaje _____ (Número de errores. Puntaje máximo = 20)

6.1 TRANSFORMACIONES GRAMATICALES: VERBOS A SUSTANTIVOS

Señale el sustantivo (la cosa) a partir del verbo (acción) (v. gr., si yo le digo jugar que es un verbo, usted me responde juego, que es un sustantivo)

1. volar _____ (vuelo)	3. enredar _____ (enredo)
2. gritar _____ (grito)	4. comer _____ (comida)

6.2 TRANSFORMACIONES GRAMATICALES: SUSTANTIVOS Y ADJETIVOS A VERBOS

Señale el verbo correspondiente a los siguientes sustantivos (v. gr., si yo le digo lectura, usted me responde leer; si yo le digo dibujo, usted me responde dibujar).

5. subida _____ (subir)	8. corte _____ (cortar)
6. pintura _____ (pintar)	9. belleza _____ (embellecer)
7. mirada _____ (mirar)	10. consideración _____ (considerar)

Señale los verbos correspondientes a los siguientes adjetivos (v. gr., si yo le digo sucio, usted me responde ensuciar; si yo le digo roto, usted me responde romper).

11. empacado _____ (empacar)	14. limpio _____ (limpiar)
12. obediente _____ (obedecer)	15. grande _____ (agrandar)
13. triste _____ (entristecer)	

6.3 TANSFORMACIONES GRAMATICALES: ANTONIMOS

Señale lo opuesto de cada una de las siguientes palabras (v. gr., si yo le digo bonito, usted me responde feo; si yo le digo interes, usted me responde desinterés).

16. gordo _____   22. visible _____
    (flaco, delgado)   (invisible)

17. pobre _____   23. normal _____
    (rico)   (anormal)

18. verdadero _____   24. real _____
    (falso)   (irreal)

19. entrar _____   25. igual _____
    (salir)   (desigual)

20. valiente _____   26. conocido _____
    (cobarde)   (desconocido)

21. vivir _____   27. rompible _____
    (morir)   (irrompible)

Puntaje ____ (Número de errores. Puntaje máximo = 27.)

7. CONSTRUCCIONES COMPARATIVAS

Responda si las siguientes afirmaciones son verdaderas (V) o falsas (F).

1. Los aviones son más rápidos que los carros   V
2. Los carros son más rápidos que los aviones.   F
3. Los aviones son más lentos que los carros.   F
4. Los carros son más lentos que los aviones.   V
5. Los aviones son menos rápidos que los carros.   F
6. Los carros son menos rápidos que los aviones.   V
7. Los aviones son menos lentos que los carros.   V
8. Los carros son menos lentos que los aviones.   F
9. Los aviones no son más rápidos que los carros.   F
10. Los carros no son más rápidos que los aviones.   V
11. Los aviones no son más lentos que los carros.   V
12. Los carros no son más lentos que los aviones.   F

Puntaje ____ (Número de respuestas incorrectas. Puntaje máximo = 12.)

8.   MANEJO DE ORACIONES COORDINADAS

Responda a las siguientes preguntas partiendo de esta afirmacion:

A. *El niño que acaricia al perro es mi hermano.*

   1. Quién acaricia al perro? _____ (el niño, mi hermano)
   2. Quién es mi hermano? _____ (el niño que acaricia al perro)
   3. Qué hace el niño? _____ (acaricia al perro)
   4. Qué hace mi hermano? _____ (acaricia al perro)
   5. A quién acaricia mi hermano? _____ (al perro)

B. *La secretaria que me enviaste con tu prima es amiga de Pedro.*

   6. Quién es amiga de Pedro _____ (la secretaria)
   7. Quién me envió la secretaria? _____ (tú)
   8. Con quién enviaste la secretaria? _____ (con tu prima)
   9. Quién es amiga de Pedro? _____ (la secretaria)
   10. De quién es amigo Pedro? _____ (de la secretaria)

   Puntaje _____ (Número de respuestas incorrectas. Puntaje máximo = 10)

Resumen de los Puntajes

1. Lenguaje espontáneo (total de palabras)   _____
2. Contrucción de frases (verbos)   _____
3. Contrucción de frases (preposiciones)   _____
4. Concordancia de artículos   _____
5. Concordancia de adjetivos   _____
6. Transformaciones gramaticales   _____
7. Construcciones comparativas   _____
8. Oraciones coordinadas   _____

Puntaje Total de Errores (2 + 3 + 4 + 5 + 6 + 7 + 8)   _____

A9. Versión Española de la Prueba de las Fichas (Token Test)

Nombre _____   Edad _____

Escolaridad _____   Fecha _____

Examinador _____

Primera Parte (se usan todas las fichas)

1. Señale un circulo
2. Señale un cuadrado
3. Señale una figura amarilla
4. Señale una figura roja
5. Señale una figura negra
6. Señale una figura verde
7. Señale una figura blanca

Segunda Parte (solamente las fichas grandes)

8. Señale un cuadrado amarillo
9. Señale un círculo negro
10. Señale un círculo verde
11. Señale un cuadrado blanco

Tercera Parte (todas las fichas)

12. Señale un círculo blanco pequeño
13. Señale el cuadrado amarillo grande
14. Señale el cuadrado verde grande
15. Señale el círculo blanco pequeño

Cuarta Parte (solamente las fichas grandes)

16. Señale el círculo rojo y el cuadrado verde
17. Señale el cuadrado amarillo y el cuadrado blanco
18. Señale el cuadrado blanco y el círculo verde
19. Señale el círculo blanco y el círculo rojo

Quinta Parte (todas las fichas)

20. Señale el círculo blanco grande y el cuadrado verde pequeño
21. Señale el círculo negro pequeño y el cuadrado amarillo grande

22. Señale el cuadrado verde grande y el cuadrado rojo grande
23. Señale el cuadrado blanco grande y el circulo verde pequeno
24. Ponga el círculo rojo sobre el cuadrado verde
25. Con el cuadrado rojo senale el circulo blanco
26. Señale el círculo blanco y el cuadrado rojo
27. Señale el círculo blanco o el cuadrado rojo
28. Ponga el cuadrado verde lejos del cuadrado amarillo
29. Si hay un círculo azul, senale el cuadrado rojo
30. Ponga el cuadrado verde al lado del círculo rojo
31. Señale los cuadrados lentamente y los círculos rapidamente
32. Ponga el círculo rojo entre el cuadrado amarillo y el cuadrado verde
33. Señale todos los circulo excepto el verde
34. Señale el círculo rojo, pero no el cuadrado blanco
35. En lugar del cuadrado blanco, señale el círculo amarillo
36. Ademas de señalar el círculo amarillo, señale el círculo negro

Sexta Parte (solamente las fichas grandes)

Puntaje total (respuestas correctas) ———————
Corrección por escolaridad y edad ———————
Puntaje corregido ———————

Corrección por edad y escolaridad para la prueba de las fichas:

	Educación (años)		
Edad	0–5	6–12	>12
16–30	3	2	0
31–50	3	3	1
51–65	4	3	2

A10. Prueba de Fluidez Verbal

Animales	Frutas	F	A	S
Total				

Total semántica _____   Promedio _____

Total fonologico _____   Promedio _____

Errores por repetición _____   Intrusiones _____

Palabras derivadas _____   Nombre propios _____

A11. Prueba de Cálculo
(use cards C-1, C2, C3, and C-4)

Nombre _____   Edad _____

Escolaridad _____   Fecha _____

Examinador _____

1. *Reading of numbers.* (Card C-1) The subject is instructed to read the following numbers, which appear on a card ("Lea los siguientes números."):

   2   7   5   27   49   94   731   3091   4908   10003

Score: Each item is scored either 0 (correct) or 1 (incorrect or impossible). Types of errors considered are (1) decomposition of numbers (inability to read a number as a unit, for example, 27 becomes 2, 7); (2) order errors (lexical substitutions: 5 becomes 6, 27 becomes 23); (3) hierarchy errors (syntactical substitutions: 27 becomes 270); (4) perseveration (repetition of the previous number); (5) inversion (digit sequence inverted: 731 becomes 713); (6) neglect (omission of left-sided digits: 731 becomes 31). Maximum score = 10.

2. *Writing of numbers.* The subject is instructed to write the following numbers to dictation ("Escriba los siguientes números."):

   3   9   4   36   58   87   642   5018   7603   20107

Score: Each item is scored either 0 (correct) or 1 (incorrect or impossible). Types of errors considered are (1) order errors; (2) hierarchy errors; (3) perseveration; (4) inversion; (5) writing of irrelevant numbers (even though the subject correctly repeats the dictated number, he or she may write a nonrelated number; (6) feature addition (writing numbers with extra strokes; (7) number addition (duplication of a number: 49 becomes 499). Maximum score = 10.

3. *Transcoding from numbers to letters.* The subject is instructed to write the corresponding word for the following written numerals ("Transcriba en letras los siguientes números."):

   8   5   9   47   382   1504   8643   10003

Score: Each item is scored 0 (correct) or 1 (incorrect or impossible). Types of errors considered are (1) decomposition (writing of digits as independent units); 15 is transcoded as one five), (2) order (15 is transcoded as sixteen); (3) hierarchy (15 is transcoded as one hundred and fifty), (4) letter omission (5) omission of grammatical particles (i.e., in Spanish the names of some numbers require the word *and*, although in English this can be omitted); (6) literal substitutions (15 is written as fifteen); (7) mixtures of codes (382 is written as 3 hundred eighty 2); (8) neglect (1504 is transcoded as five hundred and four); (9) feature omission; (10) feature addition; (11) letter addition (8 is transcoded as eighth); (12) perseveration (repetition of a former number). Maximum score = 8.

4. *Transcoding from letters to numbers.* The subject is instructed to write in front of each item the corresponding number ("Escriba los números correspondientes"):

_____ seven	_____ one hundred eighty-nine
_____ eighteen	_____ seven hundred one
_____ twenty-three	_____ one thousand eight
_____ ninety-two	_____ twelve thousand three hundred seventy-nine

Score: Each item is scored 0 (correct) or 1 (incorrect or impossible). Errors considered are (1) decomposition (twenty three is written 203); (2) order (eighteen is written 19); (3) hierarchy (eighteen is written 180); (4) perseveration (subject writes the previous number); (5) addition of numbers (ninety-two is written 192); (6) neglect (seven hundred one is written 1); (7) number omission other than neglect (one thousand eight is written 108); (8) inversions (ninety-two is written 29). Maximum score = 8.

5. *Relations "greater than" and "smaller than"* (Card C-2). Subject is instructed to indicate which number in the written pair is bigger ("mayor") or smaller ("menor"). ("Cuál de estos números es . . .")

189–201, bigger (mayor)
47–74, bigger (mayor)
36–63, smaller (menor)
3002–1967, smaller (menor)
10003–4908, smaller (menor)
3967–5102, bigger (mayor)

Score: Each item is scored 0 (correct) or 1 (incorrect). Maximum score = 6.

6. *Mental mathematical operations.* The following operations are presented orally to the subject ("Realise los siguientes operaciones aritméticas."):

$$3 + 5 = \text{_____}$$ $$55 + 38 = \text{_____}$$

$$15 - 7 = \text{_____}$$ $$93 - 13 = \text{_____}$$

$$9 \times 4 = \text{_____}$$ $$13 \times 12 = \text{_____}$$

$$9 / 3 = \text{_____}$$ $$150 / 30 = \text{_____}$$

Score: Each item is scored 0 (correct) or 1 (incorrect). Maximum score = 8.

7. *Written arithmetical operations* (Card C-3). Subject is instructed to give oral answers to the following operations, which are presented on a card ("Dé la respuesta correcta a las operaciones aritméticas escritas en esta lámina."):

3	8	9	$18 \div 3$
$+2$	-6	$\times 4$	

55	93	13	
$+38$	-61	$\times 12$	$150 \div 30$

Score: Each item is scored 0 (correct) or 1 (incorrect). Maximum score = 8.

8. *Complex written arithmetical operations.* The subject is asked to accomplish the following operations on paper, with the numbers written:

689	421	212	
$+437$	-277	$\times 324$	$818 \div 356$

Score: Each of the digits included in the right answer is scored as 0 (correct) or 1. Maximum number of possible errors is 25, following the scoring system proposed by Grafman and associates (1982). The types of errors considered are (1) confusion of arithmetical signs; (2) carrying errors (absence of carrying); (3) misplacement in carrying (carried number is wrongly located); (4) errors in column alignment (inability to write numbers in columns, either when dictated or when multiplying); (5) mixture of procedures (performing two different operations in the same task; (6) reasoning errors (impossible results, which the subject does not intend to correct: $421 - 277 = 650$.

9. *Reading of arithmetical signs* (Card C-4). The subject is asked to read the following arithmetical signs written on a card ("¿Qué signos encuentra en esta lámina?"):

$$\times \quad \div \quad - \quad + \quad =$$

Score: Each item is scored 0 (correct) or 1 (incorrect).

10. *Successive operations.* The subject is asked to continue orally the following sequence: "One plus three equals four; four plus three equals seven . . ." ("Uno más tres es igual a cuatro; cuatro más tres es igual a siete . . .") The subject must continue until 40. And "one hundred minus thirteen equal eighty seven; eighty-seven minus thirteen equals . . ." ("Cien menos trece es igual a ochenta y siete; ochenta y siete menos trece es igual a . . .") The subject must continue until 61.

$$1 \quad 4 \quad 7 \quad 10 \quad 13 \quad 16 \quad 19 \quad 22 \quad 25 \quad 28 \quad 31 \quad 34 \quad 37 \quad 40;$$
$$100 \quad 87 \quad 74 \quad 61$$

Score: Each correct response is scored 0 (correct) or 1 (wrong). Maximum score = 16.

11. *Forward and backward counting.* The patient is required to count from 1 to 20 and from 70 to 80 and backward from 20 to 1 and from 80 to 70. ("Cuente de 1 a 20; cuente hacia atrás desde 20; cuente hacia atrás de 80 a 70.")

$$1, \quad 2, \quad 3, \ldots 20$$
$$20, 19, 18, \ldots 1$$
$$70, 71, 72, \ldots 80$$
$$80, 79, 78, \ldots 70$$

Score: Each mistake in the series, including skipping a number, is scored as 0.5. Maximum score = 30.

12. *Aligning numbers in columns.* Numbers are orally presented to the patient; he is asked to write and align them as if he were going to sum them. ("Cologue en columnas, como para sumar, los siguientes números.")

$$19, 346, 501, 1709, 2, 10030$$

Score: Each number is scored 0 (correct) or 1 (incorrect). Substitutions of numbers are not penalized. Maximum score = 6.

13. *Word Problems.* The patient is asked to give the answer to the following problems presented orally ("Responda los siguientes problemas."):

1. How many apples are in one and a half dozen?
2. How many centimeters are in two and a half meters?
3. If John has 10 oranges and gives 6 away, how many remain?
4. Mary earns eight dollars per hour. How much money does she get for four hours of work?

5. Peter and Robert together have 150 dollars. Peter has the double of Robert. How much does each one have?

Score: Each right answer is scored 0 and each wrong answer 1.

Puntaje total   _____

Correción por escolaridad   _____

Puntajo corregido   _____

Laminas C-1, C-2, C-3, and C-4

2	7	5
27	49	94
731		3091
10003		4098

C-1

189--201

47--74

36--63

3002--1967

10003--4908

3967--5102

C-2

$$3$$
$$+\ 2$$

$$55$$
$$+\ 38$$

$$8$$
$$-\ 6$$

$$93$$
$$-\ 61$$

$$9$$
$$\times\ 4$$

$$13$$
$$\times\ 12$$

$$18 \div\ 3$$

$$150 \div\ 30$$

C-3

X   ÷   -   +   =

C-4

A12. Curva de Aprendizaje Verbal

Nombre _____ Edad _____

Escolaridad _____ Fecha _____

Examinador _____

	niño	perro	rosa	luna	piso	mesa	casa	cama	gato	lápiz	Total
Ensayo 1	___	___	___	___	___	___	___	___	___	___	___
Ensayo 2	___	___	___	___	___	___	___	___	___	___	___
Ensayo 3	___	___	___	___	___	___	___	___	___	___	___
Ensayo 4	___	___	___	___	___	___	___	___	___	___	___
Ensayo 5	___	___	___	___	___	___	___	___	___	___	___
Ensayo 6	___	___	___	___	___	___	___	___	___	___	___
Ensayo 7	___	___	___	___	___	___	___	___	___	___	___
Ensayo 8	___	___	___	___	___	___	___	___	___	___	___
Ensayo 9	___	___	___	___	___	___	___	___	___	___	___
Ensayo 10	___	___	___	___	___	___	___	___	___	___	___
Evocación Diferida	___	___	___	___	___	___	___	___	___	___	___

Número de palabras en el primer ensayo _____

Número de palabras en el ultimo ensayo _____

Número de ensayos requeridos _____ Intrusiones _____

Número de veces en que una palabra se repite en el mismo ensayo

_____

Tipo de curva: Productiva Improductiva Estereotipada Desorganizada

Número de palabras en memoria diferida (despues de 10–15 minutos)

A13. Prueba de Memoria Facial
(Fotografías y Hoja de Repuestas)

Answer sheet for the test of memory of unfamiliar faces

I am going to show you some pictures of unknown people. Some of them are going to be repeated. I want you to tell me whenever you see a repeated face. (Repeated faces are marked +) ("Voy a mostarte algunas fotografias de personas desconocidas. Algunas de estas totos van a aparecer repetidas. Quiero que me señale cuando aparezca una foto-grafía repetida.")

(1) _____	(2) _____	(3) _____
(4) _____	(5) _____	(6) _____
(7) _____	(13) _____	(19)+ _____
(8) _____	(14) _____	(20) _____
(9)+ _____	(15)+ _____	(21) _____
(10) _____	(16) _____	(22)+ _____
(11) _____	(17) _____	(23) _____
(12)+ _____	(18) _____	(24)+ _____

Correct recognition responses (maximum 6) _____

False positive _____

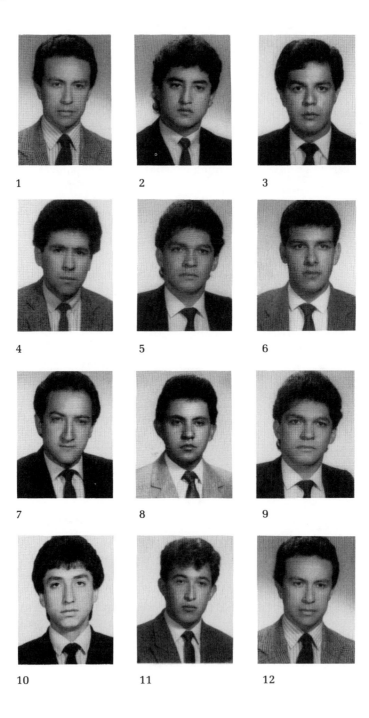

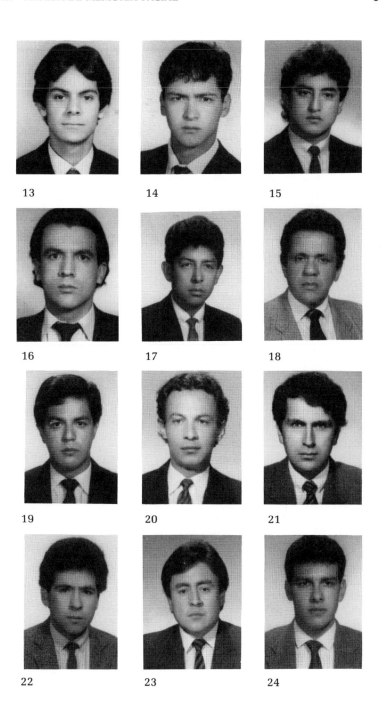

13   14   15

16   17   18

19   20   21

22   23   24

A14. Figura Compleja de Rey-Osterrieth

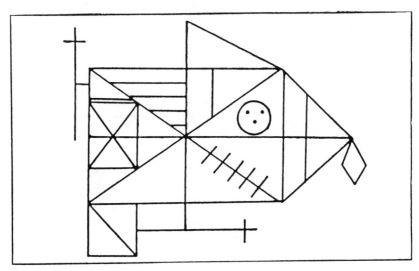

From *Archives de Psychologie* (1944), *30*, 206–356. Reprinted by permission of Editions Médecine et Hygiène, Geneva, Switzerland.

A15.   Prueba de Dibujo de un Cubo

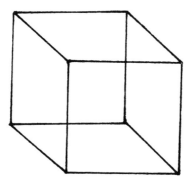

Tables of Test Norms: Percentages, Percentiles, and *T* Scores

TABLE B1. "A" Cancellation Test Norms for
Subjects of Various Ages at Two Levels (0–5 Years
and More Than 5 Years) of Formal Education

Raw scores	Percentage	Percentile	T score
Age 55 to 65 years with 0–5 years of formal education[1]			
5	4	3	21
7	6	5	28
9	8	7	34
10	15	11	38
11	18	16	41
12	21	19	44
13	35	28	47
14	46	41	51
15	52	49	54
16	100	76	57
Age 55 to 65 years with more than 5 years of formal education[2]			
10	2	2	14
11	4	3	21
12	5	5	28
13	14	10	35
14	20	17	42
15	34	27	49
16	100	67	56

(continued)

TABLE B1.   (Continued)

Raw scores	Percentage	Percentile	T score
Age over 65 years with 0–5 years of formal education[3]			
5	14	12	37
6	15	14	39
7	20	18	41
8	22	21	43
9	27	24	45
10	31	29	47
11	35	33	49
12	43	39	51
13	50	47	53
14	61	55	55
15	74	68	57
16	100	87	59
Age over 65 years with more than 5 years of formal education[4]			
9	6	5	29
10	8	7	33
11	10	9	37
12	17	13	41
13	24	20	45
14	33	28	49
15	53	43	52
16	100	76	56

[1]Mean = 13.81; SD = 3.06; range: 5–16.
[2]Mean = 15.19; SD = 1.44; range: 10–16.
[3]Mean = 11.56; SD = 4.99; range: 5–16.
[4]Mean = 14.38; SD = 2.54; range: 9–16.

TABLE B2.   Digit Symbol Test Norms for Subjects of Various Ages at Two Levels (0–5 Years and More Than 5 Years) of Formal Education

Raw score	Percentage	Percentile	T score
Age 55 to 65 years with 0–5 years of formal education[1]			
2	2	1	35
4	4	3	38
5	6	5	39
6	8	7	40
7	15	11	41
8	23	19	42
9	31	28	43
10	40	35	45
11	44	42	46
12	48	46	47
13	54	51	48
14	56	55	49
15	65	60	50
16	69	67	51
17	35	72	53
18	79	77	54
19	81	80	55
21	85	83	57
22	88	86	58
24	92	91	60
30	94	93	67
37	96	95	75
42	98	97	81
44	100	99	80

(continued)

TABLE B2.   (Continued)

Raw score	Percentage	Percentile	T score
Age 55 to 65 years with more than 5 years of formal education[2]			
4	1	1	30
7	2	2	32
8	4	4	33
15	9	7	37
17	15	13	38
18	17	16	39
19	19	18	40
20	21	20	40
21	24	22	41
22	25	24	42
23	27	26	42
24	30	29	43
25	31	31	44
26	33	32	44
27	33	35	45
28	41	39	46
30	42	41	47
32	44	43	48
33	46	45	49
34	48	47	50
35	53	50	50
36	57	55	51
37	58	58	51
38	61	60	52
39	64	63	53
40	66	65	54
41	68	67	54
42	72	70	55
43	74	73	56
44	77	76	56
45	79	78	57
47	81	80	58
49	83	82	60
50	88	85	60
52	89	88	62
55	90	89	63
56	94	93	64
60	96	95	67
65	97	96	70
67	98	97	72
70	99	98	74
75	100	99	77

TABLE B2. (Continued)

Raw score	Percentage	Percentile	T score
Age over 65 years with 0–5 years of formal education[3]			
1	14	13	39
2	21	17	40
3	24	22	41
4	29	27	42
5	36	33	43
6	40	38	45
7	46	43	46
8	50	49	47
9	54	53	48
10	56	55	49
11	57	56	50
12	58	58	52
13	61	60	53
14	64	63	54
15	71	67	55
16	76	74	56
17	79	78	57
18	82	81	59
20	85	83	61
22	89	88	63
23	90	90	64
26	93	92	68
27	97	95	69
31	100	99	74
Age over 65 years with more than 5 years of formal education[4]			
2	4	4	35
3	6	5	36
5	6	6	37
6	9	8	38
7	11	10	39
9	14	13	40
10	16	15	41
12	22	22	42

(continued)

TABLE B2. (Continued)

Raw score	Percentage	Percentile	T score
Age over 65 years with more than 5 years of formal education[4]			
13	24	23	43
15	35	32	44
16	38	36	45
17	40	39	46
18	44	42	46
19	48	46	47
20	51	50	48
21	53	52	48
22	56	55	49
23	60	58	50
24	61	60	50
25	62	61	51
26	65	63	52
27	66	65	52
28	69	67	53
29	70	69	54
30	73	72	55
32	76	75	56
33	76	76	57
35	78	77	58
36	79	78	59
37	81	80	59
38	83	82	60
39	84	84	61
41	87	86	62
42	88	87	63
43	90	89	64
45	91	90	65
46	93	92	66
48	94	93	67
51	95	94	69
53	97	96	70
54	98	97	71
59	99	98	75
60	99	99	75
73	100	99	84

[1]Mean = 14.71; SD = 8.94; range = 2–44.
[2]Mean = 34.40; SD = 14.99; range = 4–75.
[3]Mean = 10.66; SD = 8.55; range = 1–31.
[4]Mean = 23.44; SD = 14.44; range = 2–73.

TABLE B3.   Spanish Naming Test Norms for
Subjects of Various Ages at Two Levels (0–5 Years
and More Than 5 Years) of Formal Education

Raw score	Percentage	Percentile	T score
Age 55 to 65 years with 0–5 years of formal education[1]			
34	2	1	23
35	4	3	27
36	6	5	30
37	8	7	34
38	12	10	37
39	19	16	40
40	33	26	44
41	44	39	47
42	52	48	51
43	65	58	54
44	75	70	58
45	100	87	61
Age 55 to 65 years with more than 5 years of formal education[2]			
36	2	2	10
38	3	3	20
41	10	7	36
42	16	13	41
43	36	26	46
44	43	40	51
45	100	71	56

(continued)

TABLE B3.   (Continued)

Raw score	Percentage	Percentile	T score
Age over 65 years with 0–5 years of formal education[3]			
25	2	1	22
27	4	3	26
29	5	5	30
31	7	6	33
32	15	11	35
34	18	16	39
35	22	20	41
36	27	24	43
37	30	28	45
38	36	33	47
39	38	37	49
40	41	39	51
41	54	47	53
42	68	61	55
43	77	72	57
44	86	82	59
45	100	93	61
Age over 65 years with more than 5 years of formal education[4]			
33	3	2	22
34	5	4	25
35	6	5	28
36	8	7	31
37	12	10	34
38	15	14	37
39	17	15	40
40	19	18	43
41	28	24	46
42	36	32	49
43	49	43	52
44	58	54	55
45	100	79	58

[1]Mean = 41.79; SD = 2.91; range: 34–45.
[2]Mean = 43.79; SD = 1.93; range: 36–45.
[3]Mean = 39.43; SD = 5.11; range: 25–45.
[4]Mean = 42.41; SD = 3.36; range: 33–45.

TABLE B4. Verbal Fluency Test Norms for Subjects of Various Ages at Two Levels (0–5 Years and More Than 5 Years) of Formal Education

Raw score	Percentage	Percentile	T score
Age 55 to 65 years with 0–5 years of formal education			
Phonological fluency: Letter A[1]			
1	10	8	33
2	13	11	35
5	23	18	42
6	27	25	44
7	38	32	46
8	50	44	48
9	56	53	50
10	67	61	53
11	73	70	55
12	77	75	57
14	85	81	61
15	96	91	63
17	98	97	68
18	100	99	70
Phonological fluency: Letter S[2]			
1	4	3	31
2	8	6	33
3	10	9	36
4	15	13	39
5	23	19	42
6	31	27	44
7	48	40	47
8	56	52	50
9	63	59	52
10	70	67	55
11	81	76	58
12	85	83	61
13	96	91	63
14	98	97	66
17	100	99	74

(continued)

TABLE B4.   (Continued)

Raw score	Percentage	Percentile	T score
Age 55 to 65 years with 0–5 years of formal education			
Semantic fluency: Category Animals[3]			
7	4	3	36
8	8	6	38
9	17	13	40
10	35	26	43
11	40	38	45
12	44	42	47
13	50	47	50
14	60	55	52
15	69	65	54
16	75	72	57
17	90	82	59
18	92	91	61
19	94	93	64
20	96	95	66
21	98	97	68
24	100	99	75
Semantic fluency: Category Fruits[4]			
8	10	6	38
9	25	18	41
10	35	30	44
11	48	42	47
12	52	50	50
13	65	58	53
14	75	70	56
15	90	82	59
16	94	92	62
18	96	95	68
19	100	98	70

TABLE B4. (Continued)

Raw score	Percentage	Percentile	T score
Age 55 to 65 years with more than 5 years of formal education			
Phonological fluency: Letter A[5]			
1	2	2	26
3	3	3	30
4	4	4	32
5	6	5	34
6	8	7	36
7	14	11	38
8	20	17	40
9	25	22	42
10	30	28	44
11	34	32	45
12	41	38	47
13	50	45	49
14	58	54	51
15	63	60	53
16	71	67	55
17	79	75	57
18	84	81	59
19	90	87	61
20	93	91	63
21	95	94	65
22	98	96	67
23	99	98	69
24	100	99	71
Phonological fluency: Letter S[6]			
3	3	2	31
4	6	5	34
5	9	8	36
6	16	13	38
7	22	19	40
8	25	23	42
9	31	28	44
10	39	35	47
11	49	44	49
12	61	55	51
13	68	65	53
14	76	72	55
15	80	78	57
16	86	83	60
17	90	88	62

(continued)

TABLE B4.   (Continued)

Raw score	Percentage	Percentile	T score
Age 55 to 65 years with more than 5 years of formal education			
Phonological fluency: Letter S[6]			
18	94	92	64
19	95	94	66
20	97	96	68
21	98	97	71
22	90	98	73
24	100	99	77
Semantic fluency: Category Animals[7]			
6	2	2	27
9	3	3	33
10	6	5	35
11	10	8	37
12	14	12	39
13	21	17	42
14	31	26	44
15	38	34	46
16	46	42	48
17	52	49	50
18	66	59	52
19	75	70	54
20	81	78	57
21	85	83	59
22	90	88	61
23	93	91	63
24	95	94	65
25	96	95	67
26	97	96	69
28	99	98	74
29	100	99	76

TABLE B4. (Continued)

Raw score	Percentage	Percentile	T score
Age 55 to 65 years with more than 5 years of formal education			
Semantic fluency: Category Fruits[8]			
7	2	2	31
8	4	3	34
9	14	9	36
10	16	15	39
11	20	18	41
12	29	24	44
13	40	34	46
14	49	44	49
15	63	56	52
16	68	67	54
17	81	74	57
18	89	85	59
19	92	90	62
20	97	94	64
22	98	97	69
23	99	98	72
26	100	99	80
Age over 65 years with 0–5 years of formal education			
Phonological fluency: Letter A[9]			
1	8	7	35
2	12	10	38
3	23	18	40
4	32	27	43
5	40	36	45
6	47	43	48
7	56	51	50
8	62	59	53
9	73	67	55
10	84	78	58
11	85	84	60
12	90	88	63
13	96	93	65
14	97	97	67
17	100	99	75

(continued)

TABLE B4.   (Continued)

Raw score	Percentage	Percentile	T score
Age over 65 years with 0–5 years of formal education			
Phonological fluency: Letter S[10]			
1	15	11	37
2	22	18	40
3	30	26	42
4	37	34	45
5	47	42	47
6	53	50	50
7	66	60	52
8	73	69	54
9	79	76	57
10	82	81	59
11	90	86	62
12	92	91	64
13	95	93	67
14	97	96	69
15	99	98	72
17	100	99	76
Semantic fluency: Category Animals[11]			
3	1	1	29
4	4	3	31
5	5	5	34
6	12	9	37
7	16	14	39
8	23	20	42
9	32	27	45
10	48	40	47
11	56	52	50
12	64	60	53
13	81	73	55
14	86	84	58
15	90	88	61
16	93	92	63
17	95	94	66
19	97	96	71
20	99	98	74
22	100	99	79

TABLE B4. (Continued)

Raw score	Percentage	Percentile	T score
Age over 65 years with 0–5 years of formal education			
Semantic fluency: Category Fruits[12]			
4	1	1	30
5	4	3	33
6	10	7	36
7	16	13	39
8	30	23	43
9	42	36	46
10	58	50	49
11	64	61	52
12	79	72	55
13	89	84	59
14	90	90	62
15	93	92	65
16	97	95	68
18	99	98	75
21	100	99	84
Age over 65 years with more than 5 years of formal education			
Phonological fluency: Letter A[13]			
1	1	1	28
2	3	2	31
3	4	3	32
4	6	5	35
5	8	7	37
6	14	11	39
7	24	19	41
8	35	29	43
9	46	40	46
10	49	48	48
11	57	53	50
12	64	60	52
13	67	66	54
14	72	69	56
15	78	75	58
16	88	83	61
17	90	89	63
18	95	92	65
19	97	96	67
20	98	97	69
21	99	98	71
22	100	99	73

(continued)

TABLE B4. (Continued)

Raw score	Percentage	Percentile	T score

Age over 65 years with more than 5 years of formal education

Phonological fluency: Letter S[14]

Raw score	Percentage	Percentile	T score
1	1	1	30
2	4	3	32
3	7	6	35
4	11	9	37
5	16	14	39
6	23	19	42
7	31	27	44
8	44	38	46
9	56	50	49
10	66	61	51
11	73	69	54
12	79	76	56
13	83	81	58
14	88	85	61
15	90	89	63
16	91	90	65
17	93	92	66
18	96	94	70
19	99	97	72
20	100	99	74

Semantic fluency: Category Animals[15]

Raw score	Percentage	Percentile	T score
4	1	1	29
6	5	3	33
7	8	6	35
8	12	10	37
9	18	15	39
10	25	22	41
11	33	29	44
12	42	37	46
13	43	42	48
14	53	48	50
15	62	58	52
16	73	67	54
17	78	75	56
18	83	81	58
19	88	85	61
20	91	89	63
21	93	92	65
22	97	95	67

TABLE B4. (Continued)

Raw score	Percentage	Percentile	T score
Age over 65 years with 0–5 years of formal education			
Semantic fluency: Category Animals[15]			
23	98	97	69
24	99	98	71
27	99	99	77
29	100	99	82
Semantic fluency: Category Fruits[16]			
4	1	1	28
5	2	2	31
6	4	3	4
7	12	8	36
8	18	15	39
9	24	21	41
10	32	28	44
11	41	36	47
12	56	48	49
13	67	61	52
14	74	70	55
15	78	76	57
16	86	82	60
17	92	89	62
18	96	94	65
19	97	96	66
20	98	97	70
22	99	99	76
24	100	99	81

[1]Mean = 8.83; SD = 4.62; range = 1–18.
[2]Mean = 8.13.68; SD = 3.69; range = 1–17.
[3]Mean = 3.19; SD = 4.29; range = 7–24.
[4]Mean = 12.00; SD = 3.43; range = 8–19.
[5]Mean = 13.30; SD = 5.09; range = 1–24.
[6]Mean = 11.54; SD = 4.61; range = 3–24.
[7]Mean = 16.94; SD = 4.68; range = 6–29.
[8]Mean = 14.40; SD = 3.90; range = 7–26.
[9]Mean = 6.96; SD = 4.03; range = 1–17.
[10]Mean = 6.18; SD = 4.10; range = 1–17.
[11]Mean = 11.03; SD = 3.74; range = 1–17.
[12]Mean = 10.32; SD = 3.14; range = 4–21.
[13]Mean = 11.06; SD = 4.66; range = 1–22.
[14]Mean = 9.50; SD = 4.27; range = 1–20.
[15]Mean = 14.03; SD = 4.72; range = 4–29.
[16]Mean = 12.26; SD = 3.80; range = 4–24.

TABLE B5. Verbal Serial Learning Curve Norms for
Subjects of Various Ages at Two Levels (0–5 Years
and More Than 5 Years) of Formal Education

Raw score	Percentage	Percentile	T score
Age 55 to 65 years with 0–5 years of formal education			
Immediate recall (first trial)[1]			
3	8	4	34
4	50	29	43
5	79	65	53
6	94	86	63
7	100	97	72
Number of trials to criterion[2]			
3	2	1	31
4	10	6	34
5	25	17	38
6	35	30	41
8	44	40	48
10	48	46	55
11	100	74	58
Delayed memory[3]			
4	4	2	29
5	10	7	36
6	38	24	42
7	58	48	49
8	75	67	55
9	92	83	61
10	100	96	68

TABLE B5.   (Continued)

Raw score	Percentage	Percentile	T score
Age 55 to 65 years with more than 5 years of formal education			
Immediate recall (first trial)[4]			
2	1	1	26
3	9	5	34
4	35	22	41
5	58	47	49
6	85	72	56
7	96	92	64
8	100	98	72
Number of trials to criterion[5]			
2	5	3	34
3	17	11	37
4	25	21	40
5	40	32	43
6	43	41	46
8	55	53	52
9	60	58	55
10	65	63	58
11	100	82	61
Delayed memory[6]			
4	4	3	30
5	11	8	35
6	23	17	40
7	34	29	45
8	54	44	51
9	78	66	56
10	100	89	61

(continued)

TABLE B5.   (Continued)

Raw score	Percentage	Percentile	T score
Age over 65 years with 0–5 years of formal education			
Imediate recall (first trial)[7]			
1	1	2	26
2	9	5	34
3	42	26	43
4	76	59	51
5	89	82	60
6	99	94	68
7	100	99	77
Number of trials to criterion[8]			
3	3	1	18
5	5	4	27
6	14	9	32
7	18	16	36
8	20	19	41
9	22	21	46
10	24	23	50
11	100	62	55
Delayed memory[9]			
2.0	6.75	4.73	32.15
3.0	12.16	9.45	36.98
4.0	28.37	20.27	41.82
5.0	44.59	36.48	46.66
6.0	63.51	54.05	51.50
7.0	83.78	73.64	56.34
8.0	91.89	87.83	61.18
9.0	95.94	93.91	66.01
10.0	100.00	97.97	70.85
Age over 65 years with more than 5 years of formal education			
Immediate recall (first trial)[10]			
1	2	1	23
2	4	3	30
3	13	9	38
4	47	30	45

TABLE B5. (Continued)

Raw score	Percentage	Percentile	T score
Age over 65 years with more than 5 years of formal education			
Immediate recall (first trial)[10]			
5	76	61	52
6	82	84	60
7	58	95	67
8	99	99	75
9	100	99	83
Number of trials to criterion[11]			
2	1	1	30
3	10	6	34
4	24	16	37
5	31	26	40
6	37	34	44
7	42	39	47
8	49	45	49
9	51	50	53
10	55	52	56
11	100	77	59
Delayed memory[12]			
2.0	2.79	1.74	24.97
3.0	6.94	4.86	29.98
4.0	11.11	9.03	34.99
5.0	18.75	14.93	40.01
6.0	34.02	26.39	45.02
7.0	58.33	46.18	50.03
8.0	77.08	67.71	55.04
9.0	90.27	83.68	60.06
10.0	100.00	95.14	65.07

[1]Mean = 4.68; SD = 1.05; range: 3–7.
[2]Mean = 8.56; SD = 2.88; range: 3–11.
[3]Mean = 7.22; SD = 1.57; range: 4–10.
[4]Mean = 5.14; SD = 1.32; range: 2–8.
[5]Mean = 7.39; SD = 3.27; range: 2–11.
[6]Mean = 7.88; SD = 1.93; range: 4–10.
[7]Mean = 3.83; SD = 1.18; range: 1–7.
[8]Mean = 9.91; SD = 2.14; range: 3–11.
[9]Mean = 5.68; SD = 2.06; range: 2–10.
[10]Mean = 4.68; SD = 1.34; range: 1–9.
[11]Mean = 8.03; SD = 3.14; range: 2–11.
[12]Mean = 6.99; SD = 1.99; range: 2–10.

TABLE B6.   Digit Span Test Norms for Subjects
of Various Ages at Two Levels (0–5 Years and
More Than 5 Years) of Formal Education

Raw score	Percentage	Percentile	T score
Age 55 to 65 years with 0–5 years of formal education			
Digits Forward[1]			
3	6	3	32
4	56	31	44
5	85	71	56
6	100	93	68
Digits Backward[2]			
2	44	23	42
3	77	60	52
4	98	87	63
5	100	99	74
Age 55 to 65 years with more than 5 years of formal education			
Digits Forward[3]			
3	1	1	26
4	17	9	35
5	47	32	45
6	82	65	54
7	97	90	64
8	100	98	73
Digits Backward[4]			
2	12	7	35
3	42	27	44
4	84	63	53
5	94	90	63
6	100	97	72

TABLE B6. (*Continued*)

Raw score	Percentage	Percentile	T score
Age over 65 years with 0–5 years of formal education			
Digits Forward[5]			
3	9	5	36
4	66	38	46
5	86	76	56
6	99	93	66
7	100	99	76
Digits Backward[6]			
2	40	23	43
3	86	64	54
4	99	93	64
5	100	99	75
Age over 65 years with more than 5 years of formal education			
Digits Forward[7]			
3	1	1	28
4	24	12	37
5	57	41	47
6	86	72	56
7	97	92	65
8	100	99	75
Digits Backward[8]			
2	11	6	35
3	58	34	45
4	85	71	55
5	97	91	65
6	99	98	75
7	100	99	85

[1]Mean = 4.52; SD = 0.83; range: 3–7.
[2]Mean = 2.77; SD = 0.93; range: 2–5.
[3]Mean = 5.56; SD = 1.05; range: 3–8.
[4]Mean = 3.66; SD = 1.07; range: 2–6.
[5]Mean = 4.35; SD = 1.00; range: 3–7.
[6]Mean = 2.63; SD = 0.94; range: 2–5.
[7]Mean = 5.34; SD = 1.07; range: 3–8.
[8]Mean = 3.50; SD = 0.99; range: 2–7.

TABLE B7. Test of Memory for Unfamiliar
Faces Norms for Subjects of Various Ages
at Two Levels (0–5 Years and More Than 5 Years)
of Formal Education

Raw score	Percentage	Percentile	T score
Age 55 to 65 years with 0–5 years of formal education[1]			
1	8	5	28
2	15	11	35
3	19	17	41
4	42	30	47
5	65	3	53
6	100	82	59
Age 55 to 65 years with more than 5 years of formal education[2]			
2	4	3	25
3	11	8	33
4	31	21	42
5	56	44	50
6	100	78	59
Age over 65 years with 0–5 years of formal education[3]			
1	8	5	32
2	22	15	38
3	42	32	45
4	58	50	51
5	81	70	57
6	100	91	63
Age over 65 years with more than 5 years of formal education[4]			
1	2	1	21
2	7	5	29
3	17	12	37
4	38	27	44
5	67	52	52
6	100	83	60

[1]Mean = 4.50; SD = 1.62; range = 1–6.
[2]Mean = 4.95; SD = 1.17; range = 2–6.
[3]Mean = 3.87; SD = 1.60; range = 1–6.
[4]Mean = 4.70; SD = 1.27; range = 1–6.

TABLE B8.   Rey-Osterreith Complex Figure
Test Norms for Subjects of Various Ages
at Two Levels (0–5 Years and More Than 5 Years)
of Formal Education

Raw score	Percentage	Percentile	T score
Age 55 to 65 years with 0–5 years of formal education			
Copying of figure[1]			
8	6	5	33
9	10	9	35
11	12	11	37
13	15	14	39
14	17	16	40
15	21	19	41
16	23	22	43
17	25	24	43
18	29	27	45
19	35	34	46
20	42	39	47
21	46	44	48
22	48	47	49
23	53	50	50
24	56	54	51
25	60	58	54
26	62	61	55
27	73	68	55
28	75	74	56
31	79	77	59
32	85	82	60
33	88	86	62
34	90	89	63
35	96	93	64
36	100	98	65

(continued)

TABLE B8.   (Continued)

Raw score	Percentage	Percentile	T score
Age 55 to 65 years with 0–5 years of formal education			
Immediate recall[2]			
0	6	3	34
1	8	7	35
2	10	9	36
4	17	14	41
5	31	27	42
6	35	34	44
7	40	39	46
8	48	46	48
9	54	51	49
10	65	60	52
11	67	66	53
12	71	70	55
13	77	74	56
14	81	79	59
15	83	82	60
16	85	84	61
17	88	86	64
19	92	91	66
20	98	96	68
21	100	99	70
Age 55 to 65 years with more than 5 years of formal education			
Copying of figure[3]			
14	3	3	20
20	4	4	32
21	5	5	33
22	6	6	35
23	11	9	37
25	16	14	40
26	17	16	43
27	19	18	44
28	23	22	46
29	29	27	47
30	34	32	49
31	37	35	51
32	52	45	53
33	66	59	54
34	78	72	56
35	95	86	58
36	100	97	59

TABLE B8.   (Continued)

Raw score	Percentage	Percentile	T score
Age 55 to 65 years with more than 5 years of formal education			
Immediate recall[4]			
2	6	4	33
3	7	7	35
5	13	12	37
6	16	15	40
7	18	17	40
8	25	23	42
9	29	28	43
10	32	32	45
11	37	35	46
12	44	42	48
13	53	51	49
14	57	56	50
15	60	59	52
16	64	62	53
17	68	66	55
18	71	69	56
19	74	73	58
20	76	75	59
21	81	78	61
22	88	85	62
23	94	93	63
24	96	95	65
25	98	97	66
27	99	98	69
30	100	99	73
Age over 65 years with 0–5 years of formal education			
Copying of figure[5]			
1	9	9	37
2	15	14	38
3	19	18	39
4	22	21	40
5	25	25	41
6	27	26	42
7	32	30	43
8	36	35	44
9	43	41	45
10	47	47	46
11	49	48	47
12	51	50	47
15	53	52	50

(continued)

TABLE B8. (Continued)

Raw score	Percentage	Percentile	T score
Age over 65 years with 0–5 years of formal education			
Copying of figure[5]			
16	54	53	51
17	57	55	52
18	61	59	53
20	66	64	55
21	67	66	56
22	69	68	57
23	72	70	58
24	76	74	59
25	78	78	59
26	81	80	60
27	84	82	61
28	89	87	62
30	91	90	64
31	92	91	65
32	93	93	66
33	96	95	67
34	100	98	68
Immediate recall[6]			
0	24	19	42
1	31	28	43
2	45	41	45
3	58	55	47
4	68	64	49
5	73	72	52
6	74	74	53
7	76	75	56
8	80	79	58
9	85	82	59
10	88	86	61
11	91	89	64
12	92	91	67
13	95	94	69
14	96	95	70
17	99	97	77
21	100	99	85

TABLE B8.   (Continued)

Raw score	Percentage	Percentile	T score
Age over 65 years with more than 5 years of formal education			
Copying of figure[7]			
1	3	2	28
3	5	4	30
4	7	6	31
5	8	8	32
6	9	7	33
7	13	12	34
8	14	13	35
9	15	14	36
10	15	15	37
12	16	16	39
13	17	16	40
14	18	17	41
15	22	20	42
16	24	23	43
17	28	26	44
18	29	29	44
19	31	31	45
20	33	32	46
21	35	34	47
22	39	37	48
23	42	41	49
24	44	43	50
25	45	44	51
26	47	46	52
27	53	51	53
28	56	55	54
29	60	58	55
30	67	63	56
31	72	69	57
32	76	74	58
33	82	79	59
34	92	87	60
35	97	95	61
36	100	99	62

(continued)

TABLE B8. (Continued)

Raw score	Percentage	Percentile	T score
Age over 65 years with more than 5 years of formal education			
Immediate recall[8]			
0	12	10	38
1	14	13	39
2	22	20	40
3	29	27	42
4	35	33	43
5	40	39	45
6	43	42	46
7	48	47	47
8	51	50	49
9	54	53	50
10	61	59	52
11	67	66	53
12	72	70	55
13	73	72	56
14	77	75	57
15	80	80	59
16	82	81	60
17	86	85	62
18	88	87	63
19	92	91	65
20	94	93	66
21	95	94	68
22	97	96	69
24	98	97	72
25	99	98	73
27	99	99	76
28	100	99	77

[1]Mean = 22.55; SD = 8.79; range: 8–36.
[2]Mean = 9.43; SD = 5.80; range: 0–21.
[3]Mean = 30.56; SD = 5.75; range: 14–36.
[4]Mean = 13.70; SD = 6.92; range: 2–30.
[5]Mean = 14.74; SD = 10.78; range: 1–34.
[6]Mean = 4.28; SD = 4.65; range: 0–21.
[7]Mean = 23.62; SD = 10.19; range: 1–36.
[8]Mean = 8.90; SD = 6.95; range: 0–28.

TABLE B9. Finger-Tapping Test Norms for Subjects of Various Ages at Two Levels (0–5 Years and More Than 5 Years) of Formal Education

Raw score	Percentage	Percentile	T score
Age 55 to 65 years with 0–5 years of formal education			
Dominant hand[1]			
19	2	1	26
25	5	3	33
26	7	6	34
27	14	10	35
30	16	15	39
31	18	17	40
34	20	19	43
35	27	24	45
36	32	30	46
37	36	34	47
38	41	39	48
39	48	44	49
40	50	49	50
41	59	55	52
42	66	62	53
43	75	70	54
44	77	76	55
45	80	78	56
46	82	82	58
49	86	84	61
50	93	90	62
54	98	95	67
59	100	99	73
Nondominant hand[2]			
18	2	1	27
23	4	3	33
24	11	8	35
25	14	12	36
26	16	15	37
27	18	17	38
28	23	20	40
29	25	24	41
32	27	26	45
33	34	31	46
35	39	36	48
36	43	41	50
37	55	49	51

(continued)

TABLE B9.   (Continued)

Raw score	Percentage	Percentile	T score
Age 55 to 65 years with 0–5 years of formal education			
Nondominant hand[2]			
38	57	56	52
39	61	59	53
40	66	64	55
41	75	70	56
42	80	77	57
43	84	82	58
44	89	86	60
46	91	90	62
48	98	94	65
53	100	99	71
Age 55 to 65 years with more than 5 years of formal education			
Dominant Hand[3]			
21	2	2	28
25	3	3	32
27	4	4	34
28	5	5	35
29	9	7	36
32	10	9	38
33	11	10	39
34	12	11	40
35	18	15	41
36	23	20	42
37	29	26	43
38	31	30	44
39	32	32	45
40	38	35	46
41	42	40	47
42	48	45	48
43	51	49	49
44	57	54	50
45	58	58	51
46	66	62	51
47	68	67	52
48	71	69	53
50	74	73	55
51	77	76	56
53	78	78	58
54	81	80	59
55	83	82	60

TABLE B9. (Continued)

Raw score	Percentage	Percentile	T score
Age 55 to 65 years with more than 5 years of formal education			
Dominant hand[3]			
56	87	85	61
59	89	88	64
62	92	91	66
63	94	93	67
64	95	94	68
65	97	96	69
67	98	97	71
69	100	99	73
Nondominant hand[4]			
22	2	2	30
26	3	3	34
27	6	5	35
29	10	8	38
30	11	10	39
31	14	12	40
32	18	16	41
33	22	20	42
34	24	23	43
35	27	25	44
36	31	29	45
37	34	33	46
38	40	37	47
39	45	42	48
40	49	47	49
41	53	51	50
42	59	56	51
43	62	61	52
44	65	63	53
45	69	67	54
46	76	73	55
47	77	77	56
48	78	78	57
49	82	80	58
50	83	82	59
51	84	83	60
52	86	85	61
53	88	87	62
54	92	90	63
58	95	94	65

(continued)

TABLE B9. (Continued)

Raw score	Percentage	Percentile	T score
Age 55 to 65 years with more than 5 years of formal education			
Nondominant hand[4]			
59	96	95	68
60	97	96	69
62	98	97	71
64	99	98	73
69	100	99	78
Age over 65 years with 0–5 years of formal education			
Dominant hand[5]			
12	1	1	31
14	3	2	33
16	4	4	35
17	6	5	36
18	9	7	37
19	12	10	38
20	16	14	39
21	23	20	40
22	25	24	41
24	26	25	44
25	30	28	45
26	33	32	46
27	41	37	47
28	46	43	48
29	54	50	49
30	57	55	50
31	62	59	51
32	67	64	52
33	70	68	53
34	72	71	54
35	77	75	55
36	78	78	56
37	80	79	58
38	84	82	59
40	87	86	61
42	90	88	63
43	91	91	64
45	93	92	66
46	94	93	67
49	97	96	70

TABLE B9.   (Continued)

Raw score	Percentage	Percentile	T score
Age over 65 years with 0–5 years of formal education			
Dominant hand[5]			
50	99	98	72
57	100	99	79
Nondominant hand[6]			
12	1	1	32
13	3	2	33
15	4	4	35
17	10	7	37
18	14	12	38
19	16	15	39
20	22	19	40
21	25	23	41
22	30	28	42
24	35	33	44
25	39	37	46
26	42	41	47
27	43	43	48
28	48	46	49
29	52	50	50
30	59	56	51
31	62	61	52
32	65	64	53
33	71	68	54
34	72	72	55
35	75	74	56
36	78	77	57
38	83	80	59
39	84	83	60
40	86	85	62
41	88	87	63
42	91	90	64
43	93	92	65
44	94	93	66
45	96	95	67
48	97	96	70
51	99	98	73
52	100	99	74

(continued)

TABLE B9. (Continued)

Raw score	Percentage	Percentile	T score
Age over 65 years with more than 5 years of formal education			
Dominant hand[7]			
14	2	1	31
15	3	3	32
16	4	3	32
17	4	4	33
18	5	5	34
19	6	6	35
20	7	6	36
21	7	7	37
22	10	8	38
23	11	10	28
24	14	13	39
25	17	15	40
26	24	20	41
27	26	25	42
28	29	28	43
29	31	30	44
30	35	33	44
31	36	35	45
32	40	38	46
33	41	40	47
34	46	44	48
35	50	48	49
36	53	52	50
37	54	54	50
38	58	56	51
39	59	58	52
40	63	61	53
41	64	64	54
42	66	65	54
43	71	69	55
44	75	74	56
45	78	76	57
46	82	80	58
47	82	82	59
48	85	83	60
49	86	85	61
50	88	87	62
51	89	89	62
52	90	89	63
53	90	90	64
54	93	92	65

TABLE B9. (Continued)

Raw score	Percentage	Percentile	T score
Age 55 to 65 years with more than 5 years of formal education			
Dominant hand[7]			
55	95	94	66
56	96	96	67
57	98	97	67
66	99	98	75
68	99	99	77
72	100	99	80
Nondominant hand[8]			
15	2	1	32
16	4	3	33
17	4	4	34
19	6	5	36
20	8	7	37
21	10	9	38
22	13	11	38
23	17	15	39
24	21	19	40
25	24	23	41
26	26	25	42
27	31	29	43
28	33	32	44
29	38	35	45
30	40	39	46
31	41	40	47
32	43	42	48
33	49	46	49
34	54	51	50
35	58	56	51
36	59	58	52
37	62	60	53
38	67	64	54
39	69	68	55
40	71	70	55
41	77	74	56
42	79	78	57
43	82	81	58
44	84	83	59
45	85	84	60
46	86	85	61

(continued)

TABLE B9.   (Continued)

Raw score	Percentage	Percentile	T score

Age 55 to 65 years with more than 5 years of formal education

Nondominant hand[8]

Raw score	Percentage	Percentile	T score
47	89	88	62
48	90	89	63
49	92	91	64
50	93	93	65
52	95	94	67
53	96	96	68
55	97	97	70
57	98	97	72
60	99	98	74
61	99	99	75
63	100	99	77

[1]Mean $= 39.59$; $SD = 8.43$; range: 19–59.
[2]Mean $= 36.25$; $SD = 7.96$; range: 18–53.
[3]Mean $= 44.44$; $SD = 10.73$; range: 21–69.
[4]Mean $= 41.30$; $SD = 9.86$; range: 22–69.
[5]Mean $= 30.03$; $SD = 9.28$; range: 12–57.
[6]Mean $= 29.19$; $SD = 9.40$; range: 12–52.
[7]Mean $= 36.59$; $SD = 11.76$; range: 14–72.
[8]Mean $= 34.21$; $SD = 10.58$; range: 15–63.

References

Albert, M. S. (1988). Cognitive function. In M. S. Albert & M. B. Moss (Eds.), *Geriatric neuropsychology* (pp. 33–53). New York: Guilford.

Albert, M., Heller, J., & Milberg, W. (1988). Changes in naming ability with age. *Psychology and Aging, 3*, 173–178.

Albert, M., & Moss, M. (1984). The assessment of memory disorders in patients with Alzheimer's disease. In L. R. Squire & N. Butters (Eds.), *Neuropsychology of Memory*. New York: Guilford.

Alekoumbides, A., Charter, R. A., Adkins, T. G., & Seacat, G. F. (1987). The diagnosis of brain damage by the WAIS, WMS, and Reitan battery utilizing standarized scores corrected for age and education. *International Journal of Clinical Neuropsychology, 9*, 11–28.

Ardila, A. (1986). Aspectos conceptuales de la memoria. In A. Ardila, P. Montanez, & M. Rosselli (Eds.), *La memoria: Principios neuropsicologicos*. Medellin: Prensa Creativa.

Ardila, A. (1991). Errors resembling semantic paralexias in Spanish-speaking aphasics. *Brain and Language, 41*, 437–445.

Ardila, A., Montanes, P., Caro, C., Delgado, R., & Buckingham, H. W. (1989). Phonological transformations in Spanish-speaking aphasics. *Journal of Psycholinguistic Research, 18*, 163–180.

Ardila, A., & Ostrosky-Solis, F. (1988). *Lenguaje óral y escrito*. Mexico City: Trillas.

Ardila, A., & Rosselli, M. (1986). *La vejez: Neuropsicologia del fenomeno del envejecimiento*. Medellin: Prensa Creativa.

Ardila, A., & Rosselli, M. (October, 1988). *Effects of educational level on linguistic abilities*. Paper presented at Eighth Annual Meeting of the National Academy of Neuropsychologists, Orlando, FL.

Ardila, A., & Rosselli, M. (1989). Neuropsychological characteristics of normal aging. *Developmental Neuropsychology, 5*, 307–320.

Ardila, A., Rosselli, M., & Pinzon, O. (1989). Alexia and agraphia in Spanish speakers: CAT correlations and interlinguistic analysis. In A. Ardila & F. Ostrosky (Eds.), *Brain organization of language and cognitive processes* (pp. 147–175). New York: Plenum.

Ardila, A., Rosselli, M., & Rosas, P. (1989). Neuropsychological assessment in illiterates: Visuospatial and memory abilities. *Brain and Cognition, 11*, 147–166.

Ardila, A., & Rosselli, M. (1992). *Neuropsicología clinica*. Medellin: Prensa Creativa.

185

Avila, R. (1976). *Cuestionario para el estudio linguistico de las afasias.* Mexico City: El Colegio de Mexico.

Badcock, K. A., & Ross, M. W. (1982). Neuropsychological testing with Australian aborigines. *Australian Psychologist, 17*(3), 297–299.

Basso, A., Casati, G., & Vignolo, L. A. (1977). Phonemic identification defect in aphasia. *Cortex, 13*, 85–95.

Bauer, R. M., & Rubens, A. B. (1985). Agnosia. In K. M. Heilman & E. Valenstein (Eds.), *Clinical neuropsychology* (2nd ed.; pp. 187–242). New York: Oxford University Press.

Bayles, K. A. (1982). Language function in senile dementia. *Brain and Language, 16*, 265–280.

Benson, D. F. (1977). The third alexia. *Archives of Neurology, 34*, 327–331.

Benson, D. F. (1979). *Aphasia, alexia and agraphia.* New York: Churchill Livingston.

Benson, D. F. (1985). Alexia, In J. A. M. Frederiks (Ed.), *Handbook of clinical neurology: Vol 45. Clinical neuropsychology* (pp. 433–455). Amsterdam: Elsevier.

Benson, D. F., & Ardila, A. (in press). *Aphasia: A clinical perspective.* New York: Oxford University Press.

Benson, D. F., & Cummings, J. L. (1985). Agraphia. In J. A. M. Frederiks (Ed.), *Handbook of Clinical Neurology: Vol 45. Clinical Neuropsychology* (pp. 457–471). Amsterdam: Elsevier.

Benson, D. F., & Denckla, M. B. (1969). Verbal paraphasia as a source of calculation disturbance. *Archives of Neurology, 21*, 96–102.

Benson, D. F., Sheretana, W. A., Bouchard, R., Segarra, J. M., Price, D., & Geschwind, N. (1973). Conduction aphasia: A clinicopathological study. *Archives of Neurology, 28*, 339–346.

Benton A. L. (1967). Constructional apraxia and the mirror hemisphere. *Confinin. Neurologica, 22*, 141–155.

Benton, A. L. (1968). Differential behavioral effects in frontal lobe disease. *Neuropsychologia, 6*, 53–60.

Benton, A. L., & Hamsher, K. S. (1976). *Multilingual Aphasia Examination.* Iowa City: University of Iowa.

Benton, A. L., Hamsher, K. S., Varney, N. R., & Spreen, O. (1983). *Contributions to neuropsychological assessment: A clinical manual.* New York: Oxford University Press.

Berger, H. (1926). Uber Rechenstorunger bei Herderkraunkunger des Grosshirns. *Archive fur psychiatrie und nervenkrankheiten, 78*, 236–263.

Bernard, L. C. (1989). Halstead-Reitan Neuropsychological Test performance of Black, Hispanic, and White young adult males from poor academic backgrounds. *Archives of Clinical Neuropsychology, 4*(3), 267–274.

Binder, L. M. (1982). Constructional strategies on complex figure drawings after unilateral brain damage. *Journal of Clinical Neuropsychology, 4*, 51–58.

Black, F. W., & Strub, R. L. (1978). Digit repetition performance in patients with focal brain damage. *Cortex, 14*, 12–21.

Bleecker, M. L., Bolla-Wilson, K., Kawas, C., & Agnew, J. (1988). Age-specific norms for the Mini–Mental State Examination. *Neurology, 38*, 1565–1568.

Blumstein, S. E., Baker, E., & Goodglass, H. (1977). Phonological factors in auditory comprehension in aphasia. *Neuropsychologia, 15*, 19–30.

Bogen, J. E. (1985). The callosal syndromes. In K. M. Heilman & E. Valenstein (Eds.), *Clinical neuropsychology* (2nd ed.; pp. 295–338). New York: Oxford University Press.

Boller, F., & Grafman, J. (1983). Acalculia: Historical development and current significance. *Brain and Cognition, 2,* 205–223.

Boller, F., & Grafman, J. (1985). Acalculia. In J. A. M. Frederiks (ed.), *Handbook of clinical neurology, Vol. 45. Clinical neuropsychology.* Amsterdam: Elsevier.

Boller, F., & Vignolo, L. A. (1966). Latent sensory aphasia in hemisphere-damaged patients: An experimental study with the Token Test. *Brain, 89,* 815–831.

Bornstein, R. A. (1986). Classification rates obtained with "standard" cut-off scores on selected neuropsychological measures. *Journal of Clinical and Experimental Neuropsychology, 8,* 413–420.

Borod, J. C., Goodglass, H., & Kaplan, E. (1980). Normative data on the Boston Diagnostic Aphasia Examination and the Boston Naming Test. *Journal of Clinical Neuropsychology, 2,* 209–215.

Botwinick, J., & Storandt, M. (1974). *Memory, related functions and age.* Springfield, IL: Thomas.

Botwinick, J., Storandt, M., & Berg, L. (1986). A longitudinal, behavioral study of senile dementia of the Alzheimer type. *Archives of Neurology, 43,* 1124–1127.

Brandt, J. (1984). Clinical correlates of dementia and disability in Huntington's disease. *Journal of Clinical Neuropsychology, 6,* 401–412.

Brown, J. W. (1975). The problem of repetition: A case study of "conduction" aphasia and the "isolation" syndrome. *Cortex, 11,* 37–52.

Bruyer, R. (1986). Face processing and brain damage: Group studies. In R. Bruyer (Ed.), *The neuropsychology of face perception and facial expression.* Hillsdale, NJ: Erlbaum.

Caplan, D., Vanier, M., & Baker, C. (1986). A case study of reproduction conduction aphasia: I. Word production. *Cognitive Neuropsychology, 3,* 99–128.

Caramazza, A., Basili, A. G., Koller, J. J., & Berndt, R. S. (1981). An investigation of repetition and language processing in a case of conduction aphasia. *Brain and Language, 14,* 235–271.

Caramazza, A., & McClosky, M. (1987). Dissociations of calculation processes. In G. Deloche & X. Seron (Eds.), *Mathematical disabilities: A cognitive neuropsychological perspective* (pp. 221–234). Hillsdale, NJ: Erlbaum.

Collins, M. (1986). *Diagnosis and treatment of global aphasia.* San Diego: College-Hill Press.

Corrigan, J. D., & Hinkeldey, N. S. (1987). Comparison of intelligence and memory in patients with diffuse and focal injury. *Psychological Reports, 60,* 899–906.

Costa, L. D. (1975). The relation of the visuospatial dysfunction to Digit Span performance in patients with cerebral lesions. *Cortex, 11,* 31–36.

Crockett, D., Bilsker, D., Hurwitz, T., & Kozak, J. (1986). Clinical utility of three measures of frontal lobe dysfunction in neuropsychiatric patients. *International Journal of Neuroscience, 30,* 241–248.

Cummings, J. L., & Benson, D. F. (1983). *Dementia: A clinical approach.* Boston: Buttersworths.

Curry, J. F., Logue, P. E., & Butler, B. (1986). Child and adolescent norms for Russell's revision of the Wechsler Memory Scale. *Journal of Clinical Child Psychology, 15,* 214–220.

Dahmen, W., Hartje, W., Bussing, A., & Strum, W. (1982). Disorders of calculation in aphasic patients: Spatial and verbal components. *Neuropsychologia, 20,* 145–153.

Dalen, K., & Hugdahl, K. (1988). Hemisphere, asymmetry and finger tapping in right-handed females. *International Journal of Neuroscience, 38,* 321–329.

Damasio, A. R., & Damasio, H. (1986). The anatomical substrate of prosopagnosia. In R. Bruyer (Ed.), *The neuropsychology of face perception and facial expression*. Hillsdale, NJ: Erlbaum.

Damasio, A. R., Damasio, H., & Van Hoesen, G. W. (1982). Prosopagnosia: Anatomical bases and behavioral mechanisms. *Neurology, 32*, 331–341.

Damasio, H., & Damasio, A. (1980). The anatomical basis of conduction aphasia. *Brain, 103*, 337–350.

Damasio, H., & Damasio, A. (1983). Localization of lesions in conduction aphasia. In A. Kertesz (Ed.), *Localization in neuropsychology* (pp. 231–244). New York: Academic Press.

D'Amato, M. R. (1970). *Experimental psychology: Methodology, psychophysics and methods*. New York: McGraw-Hill.

Dejerine, S. (1892). Contribution a l'étude anatomopatholigique et clinique des différents variétés de cécité verbale. *Memoires Societé Biologie, 4*, 61–90.

D'Elia, L. F., Satz, P., & Schretlen, D. (1989). The Wechsler Memory Scale: A critical appraisal of the normative studies. *Journal of Clinical and Experimental Neuropsychology, 1*, 551–568.

Deloche, G., & Seron, X. (1984). Some linguistic aspects of calculia. In F. C. Rose (Ed.), *Advances in neurology, progress in aphasiology* (Vol. 42). New York: Raven Press.

Deloche, G., & Seron, X. (1987). Numerical transcoding: A general production model. In G. Deloche & X. Seron (Eds.), *Mathematical disabilities: A cognitive neuropsychological perspective* (pp. 137–170). Hillsdale, NJ: Erlbaum.

Deregowski, J. B. (1986). Kazimierz Bartel's observations on drawing of children and illiterate adults. *British Journal of Developmental Psychology, 4*, 331–333.

De Renzi, E., & Faglioni, P. (1978). Normative data and screening power of a shortened version of the Token Test. *Cortex, 14*, 327–342.

De Renzi, E., Faglioni, P., & Spinnler, H. (1968). The performance of patients with unilateral brain damage on face recognition tasks. *Cortex, 4*, 17–34.

De Renzi, E., & Spinnler, H. (1966). Facial recognition in brain-damaged patients: An experimental approach. *Neurology, 16*, 145–152.

De Renzi, E., & Vignolo, L. A. (1962). The Token Test: A sensitive test to detect disturbances in aphasics. *Brain, 85*, 665–678.

Dergan, J. J. (1987). La Bateria Neuropsicologica Luria-Nebraska (The Luria-Nebraska Neuropsychological Battery). *Avances en Psicologia Clinica Latinoamericana, 5*, 27–36.

Dodrill, C. B. (1979). Sex differences on the Halstead-Reitan Neuropsychological Battery and on other neuropsychological measures. *Journal of Clinical Psychology, 35*, 236–241.

Donias, S. H., Vassi Lopoulou, E. O., Golden, C. J., & Lovell, M. R. (1989). Reliability and clinical effectiveness of the standardized Greek version of the Luria-Nebraska Neuropsychological Battery. *International Journal of Clinical Neuropsychology, 11*(13), 129–133.

Escobar, J. I., Burman, A., Karno, M., Forsythe, A., Landsverk, J., & Golding, J. M. (1986). Use of the Mini–Mental State Examination (MMSE) in a community population of mixed ethnicity. *Journal of Nervous and Mental Disease, 174*, 607–614.

Farber, J. F., Schmitt, F. A., & Logue, P. E. (1988). Predicting intellectual level from the Mini–Mental State Examination. *Journal of the American Geriatrics Society, 36*, 509–510.

Faust, D. (1991). Clinical neuropsychology: Practicing a science that does not yet exist. *Neuropsychology Review*, *2*(3), 205–232.

Ferro, J. M., & Botelho, M. H. (1980). Alexia for arithmetical signs: A cause of disturbed calculation. *Cortex*, *16*, 175–180.

Finlayson, M. A. J., & Reitan, R. M. (1980). Effects of lateralized lesions on ipsolateral and contralateral motor functioning. *Journal of Clinical Neuropsychology*, *2*, 237–243.

Folstein, M. F., Folstein, S. E., & McHugh, P. R. (1975). "Mini–Mental State." *Journal of Psychiatric Research*, *12*, 189–198.

Folstein, N., Anthony, J. C., Parhad, I., Duffy, B., & Gruenberg, E. M. (1985). The meaning of cognitive impairment in the elderly. *Journal of the American Geriatrics Society*, *33*, 228–235.

Freeman, N. H. (1986). How should a cube be drawn? *British Journal of Developmental Psychology*, *4*, 317–322.

Freeman, N. H. (1987). Current problems in the development of representational picture production. *Archives of Psychologie*, *55*, 127–152.

Gainotti, G. (1985). Constructional apraxia. In J. A. M. Fredericks (Ed.), *Handbook of Clinical Neurology: Vol. 45. Clinical Neuropsychology*. Amsterdam: Elsevier.

Garcia-Albea, J. E., Sanchez-Bernardos, M. L., & del Viso-Pabon, S. (1986). Test de Boston para el diagnostico de la afasia: Adaptacion Española. In H. Goodglass & E. Kaplan (Eds.), *La evaluación de la afasia y de transtornos relacionados* (2a edicion; Carlos Wernicke, Trans.). Madrid: Editorial Medica Panamericana.

Gazzaniga, M. S., Glass, A. A., Sarno, M. T., & Posner, J. B. (1973). Pure word deafness and hemispheric dynamics: A case history. *Cortex*, *9*, 136–143.

Geschwind, N. (1975). The apraxias: Neural mechanisms of disorders of learned movements. *Scientific American*, *63*, 188–195.

Goodglass, H., Fodor, I. G., & Schulhoff, C. (1967). Prosodic factors in grammar: Evidence from aphasia. *Journal of Speech Research*, *10*, 5–16.

Goodglass, H., & Huner, M. (1970). A linguistic comparison of speech and writing in two types of aphasia. *Journal of Communication Disorders*, *3*, 28–41.

Goodglass, H., & Kaplan, E. (1972). *The assessment of aphasia and related disorders*. Philadelphia: Lea & Febiger.

Goodglass, H., & Kaplan, E. (1979). *Evaluación de la afasia y de transtornos similares* (Silvia Cuschnir de Fairman, Trans.). Buenos Aires: Editorial Médica Panamericana.

Goodglass, H., & Kaplan, E. (1983). *The assessment of aphasia and related disorders* (2nd ed.). Philadelphia: Lea & Febiger.

Goodglass, H., Klein, H., Carey, P., & Jones, K. J. (1966). Specific semantic word categories in aphasia. *Cortex*, *2*, 74–89.

Goodglass, H., Quafasel, F. A., & Timberlake, W. H. (1964). Phrase length and the type and severity of aphasia. *Cortex*, *1*, 133–140.

Grewel, F. (1960). The acalculias. In P. J. Vinken & G. W. Bruyn (Eds.), *Handbook of Clinical Neurology* (vol. 4; pp. 181–196). Amsterdam: Elsevier.

Halland, K. Y., Linn, R. T., Hunt, W. C., & Goodwin, J. S. (1983). A normative study of Russell's variant of the Wechsler Memory Scale in a healthy elderly population. *Journal of Consulting and Clinical Psychology*, *51*, 878–881.

Halstead, W. C. (1947). *Brain and intelligence*. Chicago: University of Chicago Press.

Harley, J. P., Leuthold, C. A., Matthews, C. G., & Bergs, L. E. (1980). *Wisconsin neuropsychological test battery T score norms for older veterans administration medical center patients*. Madison, WI: Matthews.

Hécaen, H., Algelergues, T., & Houiller, S. (1961). Les variétés cliniques des acalculies au cours des lesions retrorolandiques. *Revue Neurologique, 105,* 85–103.

Hécaen, H., & Ruel, J. (1981). Sieges, lesionnels intrafrontaux et deficits au test de "fluence verbale." *Revue de Neurologie, 137,* 277–284.

Henschen, S. E. (1920). *Klinische und Pathologische Beitrage zur Pathologie des Gehirn.* Stockholm: Nordiska Bokhandeln.

Hightower, M. G., & Anderson, R. P. (1986). Memory evaluation of alcoholics with Russell's revised Wechsler Memory Scale. *Journal of Clinical Psychology, 42,* 1000–1005.

Howes, D. H. (1967). Hypotheses concerning the functions of the language mechanisms. In K. Salzinger and S. Salzinger (Eds.), *Research in verbal behavior and some neurophysiological implications* (pp. 429–455). New York: Academic Press.

Huff, F. J., Collins, C., Corkin, S., & Rosen, T. J. (1986). Equivalent forms of the Boston Naming Test. *Journal of Clinical and Experimental Neuropsychology, 8,* 556–562.

Ikeda, K. (1987). Lateralized interference effects of concurrent verbal tasks on sequential finger tapping. *Neuropsychologia, 25,* 453–456.

Jackson, M., & Warrington, E. K. (1986). Arithmetic skills in patients with unilateral cerebral lesions. *Cortex, 22,* 611–622.

Kafonek, S., Ettinger, W. H., Roca, R., Kittner, S., Taylor, N., & German, P. S. (1989). Instruments for screening for depression and dementia in a long-term care facility. *Journal of the American Geriatrics Association, 32,* 29–34.

Kaplan, E. (1988). A process approach to neuropsychological assessment. In T. Boll & B. K. Bryant (Eds.), *Clinical neuropsychology and brain function: Research, measurement and practice* (pp. 127–167). Washington, DC: American Psychological Association.

Kaplan, E., Goodglass, H., & Weintraub, S. (1978). *The Boston Naming Test.* Boston: E. Kaplan & H. Goodglass.

Kean, L. M. (Ed.). (1985). *Agrammatism.* New York: Academic Press.

Kertesz, A. (1979). *Aphasia and associated disorders.* New York: Grune & Stratton.

Kertesz, A. (1983). Localization of lesions in Wernicke's aphasia. In A. Kertesz (Ed.), *Localization in neuropsychology* (pp. 209–230). New York: Academic Press.

Kertesz, A. (1985). Aphasia. In J. A. M. Frederiks (Ed.), *Handbook of clinical Neurology: Clinical neuropsychology* (vol. 45; pp. 287–331). Amsterdam: Elsevier.

Kertesz, A. (1986). Assessment of aphasia. In T. Incagnoli, G. Goldstein, & C. J. Golden (Eds.), *Clinical applications of neuropsychological test batteries* (pp. 329–360). New York: Plenum.

Kindlon, D. J., & Garrison, W. (1984). The Boston Naming Test: Norms data and cue utilization in a sample of normal 6- and 7-year-old children. *Brain and Language, 21,* 255–259.

Kleist, K. (1912). Der Gang und der gagenwurtige Stand der Apraxie-Forschung. *Ergebnisse der neurologie und psychiatrie, 1,* 342–352.

Knesevich, J. W., LaBarge, E., & Edwards, D. (1986). Predictive value of the Boston Naming Test in mild senile dementia of the Alzheimer type. *Psychiatry Research, 19,* 155–161.

Knopman, D. S., Selnes, O. A., Niccum, N., & Rubens, A. B. (1984). Recovery of naming in aphasia: Relationship to fluency, comprehension and CT findings. *Neurology, 34,* 1461–1470.

Kohn, S. E., & Goodglass, H. (1985). Picture-naming in aphasia. *Brain and Language, 24,* 266–283.

Kokmen, E., Naessens, J. M., & Offord, K. P. (1987). A short test of mental status: Description and preliminary results. *Mayo Clinic Proceedings, 62*, 281–288.

LaBarge, E., Edwards, D., & Knesevich, J. W. (1986). Performance of normal elderly on the Boston Naming Test. *Brain and Language, 24*, 380–384.

Lange, J. (1936). Agnosien and apraxien. In O. Bumke & O. Foester (Eds.), *Handbuch der Neurologie* (vol. 1; pp. 807–860). Berlin: Springer-Verlag.

Larrebee, G. J., Kane, R. L., & Schunck, J. R. (1983). Factor analysis of the WAIS and the Wechsler Memory Scale: An analysis of the construct validity of the Wechsler Memory Scale. *Journal of Clinical Neuropsychology, 5*, 159–168.

LaRue, A. (1992). *Aging and neuropsychological assessment*. New York: Plenum.

Lecours, A. R., Trepagnier, C., Naesser, C. J., & Lavelle-Huynh, G. (1983). The interaction between linguistics and aphasiology. In A. R. Lecours, F. Lhermitte, & B. Bryans (Eds.), *Aphasiology*. London: Bailliere Tindall.

Levin, H., & Spiers, P. A. (1985). Acalculia. In K. M. Heilman & E. Valenstein (Eds.), *Clinical Neuropsychology* (2nd ed.; pp. 97–114). New York: Oxford University Press.

Lezak, M. D. (1988). *Neuropsychological assessment* (2nd ed.). New York: Oxford University Press.

Liepmann, H., & Storck, E. (1902). Ein Fall von reiner Sprachtaubheit. *Manuschfrift Psychiatrie und Neurologie, 17*, 289–311.

Logue, P., & Wyrick, L. (1979). Initial validation of Russell's revised Wechsler Memory Scale: A comparison of normal aging versus dementia. *Journal of Consulting and Clinical Psychology, 47*, 176–178.

Luria, A. R. (1964). Factors and forms of aphasia. In A. V. S. De Reuck & M. O'Connor (Eds.), *Disorders of language*. London: Churchill.

Luria, A. R. (1966). *Higher cortical functions in man*. New York: Basic Books.

Luria, A. R. (1970). *Traumatic aphasia*. The Hague: Mouton.

Luria, A. R. (1973).*The working brain: An introduction to neuropsychology*. New York: Basic Books.

Luria, A. R. (1975). *The neuropsychological investigation*. Moscow: Moscow University Press (Russian).

Luria, A. R. (1976a). *Basic problems of neurolinguistics*. The Hague: Mouton.

Luria, A. R. (1976b). *The neuropsychology of memory*. Washington, D.C.: Winston.

Magaziner, J., Bassett, S. S., & Hebel, R. (1987). Predicting performance on the Mini–Mental State Examination. *Journal of the American Geriatrics Society, 35*, 996–1000.

Margolis, R. B., & Scialfa, C. T. (1984). Age differences in Wechsler Memory Scale performance. *Journal of Clinical Psychology, 40*, 1442–1449.

Marshall, J. C., & Newcombe, F. (1973). Patterns of paralexias: A psycholinguistic approach. *Journal of Psycholinguistic Research, 2*, 175–199.

Martin, A., & Fedio, P. (1983). Word-production and comprehension in Alzheimer disease: The breakdown of semantic knowledge. *Brain and Language, 19*, 124–141.

McCloskey, M., & Caramazza, A. (1987). Cognitive mechanisms in normal and impaired number processing. In G. Deloche & X. Seron (Eds.), *Mathematical disabilities: A cognitive neuropsychological perspective* (pp. 201–219). Hillsdale, NJ: Erlbaum.

McFie, J., & Zangwill, O. L. (1960). Visual-constructive disabilities associated with lesions of the right cerebral hemisphere. *Brain, 83*, 243–260.

Messerli, P., Seron, X., & Tissot, R. (1979). Quelques aspects des troubles de la programmation dans le syndrome frontal. *Archives Suisse de Neurologie, Neurochirurgie et de Psychiatrie, 125*, 23–35.

Mesulam, M. M. (1985). *Principles of behavioral neurology.* Philadelphia: Davis.

Miceli, G., Gainotti, G., Caltagirone, C., & Masullo, C. (1980). Some aspects of phonological impairment in aphasia. *Brain and Language, 11,* 159–169.

Miller, E. (1977). *Abnormal aging: The psychology of senile dementia.* New York: Wiley.

Miller, E., & Hague, F. (1975). Some characteristics of verbal behavior in presenile dementia. *Psychological Medicine, 5,* 255–259.

Milner, B. (1968). Visual recognition and recall after right temporal lobe excision in man. *Neuropsychologia, 6,* 191–209.

Murri, L., Arena, R., Siciliano, G., Mazzotta, R., & Muratorio, A. (1984). Face recall in patients with focal cerebral lesion. *Archives of Neurology, 41,* 183–185.

Nelson, A., Fogel, B. S., & Faust, D. (1986). Bedside cognitive screening instruments: A critical assessment. *Journal of Nervous and Mental Disease, 174,* 73–83.

Newcombe, F. (1969). *Missile wounds of the brain: A study of psychological deficits.* London: Oxford University Press.

Osterrieth, P. A. (1944). Le test de copie d'une figure complexe. *Archives de Psychologie, 30,* 206–356.

Piercy, M., Hecaen, H., & Ajuriaguerra, J. (1960). Constructional apraxia associated with unilateral cerebral lesions: Left- and right-sided cases compared. *Brain, 83,* 225–242.

Pillon, B. (1981). Negligence de l'hemi-espace gauche dans des preuves visuoconstructives. *Neuropsychologia, 19,* 317–320.

Prigatano, G. P. (1978). Wechsler Memory Scale: A selective review of the literature. *Journal of Clinical Psychology, 34,* 816–832.

Puente, A. E. (1990). Psychological assessment of minority group members. In G. Goldstein & M. Hersen (Eds.), *Handbook of psychological assessment* (pp. 505–520). New York: Pergamon Press.

Puente, A. E., & McCaffrey, R. J. (1992). *Handbook of neuropsychological assessment: A biopsychosocial perspective.* New York: Plenum Press.

Reitan, R., & Wolfson, D. (1985). *The Halstead-Reitan Neuropsychological Test Battery: Theory and clinical interpretation.* Tucson, AZ: Neuropsychology Press.

Rey, A. (1941). L'examen psychologique dans les cas l'encephalopathie traumatic. *Archives de Psychologie, 28,* 286–340.

Roeltgen, D. (1985). Agraphia. In K. M. Heilman & E. Valenstein (Eds.), *Clinical neuropsychology* (2nd ed.; pp. 75–96). New York: Oxford University Press.

Rosen, W. G. (1980). Verbal fluency in aging and dementia. *Journal of Clinical Neuropsychology, 2,* 135–146.

Rosen, W. G. (1983). Clinical and neuropsychological assessment of Alzheimer disease. In R. Mayeux & W. G. Rosen (Eds.), *Advances in neurology: Vol. 38. The dementias* (pp. 51–64). New York: Raven Press.

Rosselli, M., & Ardila, A. (1989). Calculation deficits in patients with right and left hemisphere damage. *Neuropsychologia, 27,* 607–617.

Rosselli, M., Ardila, A., Florez, A., & Castro, C. (1990). Normative data on the Boston Diagnostic Aphasia Examination in a Spanish-speaking population. *Journal of Clinical and Experimental Neuropsychology, 12,* 313–322.

Rosselli, M., Ardila, A., & Rosas, P. (1990). Neuropsychological assessment in illiterates: II. Language and praxic abilities. *Brain and Cognition. 12(2),* 281–296.

Rosselli, M., & Ardila, A. (1991). Effects of age, education and gender on the Rey-Osterrieth complex figure. *The Clinical Neuropsychologist, 5,* 370–376.

Russell, E. W. (1975). A multiple scoring method for the assessment of complex memory functions. *Journal of Consulting and Clinical Psychology, 43,* 800–908.

Russell, E. W. (1988). Renorming Russell's version of the Wechsler Memory Scale. *Journal of Clinical and Experimental Neuropsychology, 10*, 235–249.

Sasanuma, S., & Fujimura, O. (1971). Kanji versus Kana processing in alexia with transient agraphia: A case report. *Cortex, 7*, 1–17.

Savash, R. D., Britton, P. G., Bolton, N., & Hall, E. H. (1973). *Intellectual functioning in the aged*. New York: Harper & Row.

Shallice, T., & Warrington, E. K. (1977). Auditory-verbal short term memory impairment and conduct aphasia. *Brain and Language, 4*, 479–491.

Skelton-Robinson, M., & Jores, S. (1984). Nominal dyphasia in the severity of senile dementia. *British Journal of Psychiatry, 145*, 168–171.

Smith, S., Butters, N., White, R., & Lyon, L. (1988). Priming semantic relations in patients with Huntington's disease. *Brain and Language, 33*, 27–40.

Spellacy, F. J., & Spreen, O. (1969). A short form of the Token Test. *Cortex, 5*, 390–397.

Spitz, H. H. (1972). Note on immediate memory for digits: Invariance over the years. *Psychological Bulletin, 68*, 183–185.

Spreen, O., & Benton, A. L. (1969). *Neurosensory center comprehensive examination for aphasia*. Victoria, BC: Neuropsychological Laboratory, Department of Psychology, University of Victoria.

Statistical Abstract of the United States (110th ed.). (1990). Washington, DC: Bureau of Census.

Strub, R. L., & Black, F. W. (1981). *Neurobehavioral disorders: A clinical approach*. Philadelphia: Davis.

Stuss, D. T. (1986). Language functioning after bilateral prefrontal leukotomy. *Brain and Language, 28*, 66–70.

Stuss, D. T., & Benson, D. F. (1986). *The frontal lobes*. New York: Raven Press.

Talland, G. A. (1965). *Deranged memory*. New York: Academic Press.

Taylor, E. M. (1959). *The appraisal of children with cerebral deficits*. Cambridge, MA: Harvard University Press.

Taylor, L. B. (1969). Localization of cerebral lesions by psychological testing. *Clinical Neurosurgery, 16*, 269–287.

Terman, L. M., & Merrill, M. A. (1973). *Stanford-Binet Intelligence Scale Manual* (3rd Rev.). Boston: Houghton Mifflin.

Van-Gorp, W. G., Satz, P., Kiersch, M. E., & Henry, R. (1986). Normative data on the Boston Naming Test for a group of normal older adults. *Journal of Clinical and Experimental Neuropsychology, 8*, 702–705.

Varney, N. R., & Benton, A. L. (1979). Phonemic discrimination and aural comprehension among aphasic patients. *Journal of Clinical Neuropsychology, 1*, 65–73.

Vinarskaya, E. N. (1971). *Clinical problems of aphasia*. Moscow: Meditsina (in Russian).

Waber, D. P., & Holmes, J. M. (1985). Assessing children's copy production of the Rey-Osterrieth complex figure. *Journal of Clinical and Experimental Neuropsychology, 7*, 264–280.

Wallace, J. L. (1984). Wechsler Memory Scale. *International Journal of Clinical Neuropsychology, 6*, 216–226.

Walsh, K. (1987). *Neuropsychology: A clinical approach* (2nd ed.). Edinburgh: Churchill Livingstone.

Warrington, E. K. (1982). The fractionation of arithmetical skills: A single case study. *Journal of Experimental Psychology, 34A*, 31–51.

Warrington, E. K., & James, M. (1967). An experimental investigation of facial recognition in patients with unilateral cerebral lesion. *Cortex, 3*, 317–326.

Wechsler, D. (1945). A standardized memory scale for clinical use. *Journal of Psychology, 19*, 87–95.

Wechsler, D. (1955). *Wechsler Adult Intelligence Scale: Manual*. New York: Psychological Corporation.

Wechsler, D. (1974). *Wechsler Intelligence Scale for Children: Revised Manual*. San Antonio: The Psychological Corporation.

Wechsler, D. (1985). *Wechsler Intelligence Scale: Revised manual*. San Antonio, TX: The Psychological Corporation.

Wechsler, D. (1987). *Wechsler Memory Scale: Revised manual*. San Antonio, TX: The Psychological Corporation.

Weinberg, J., Diller, L., Gerstman, L., & Schulman, P. (1972). Digit span in right and left hemiplegics. *Journal of Clinical Psychology, 28*, 361–369.

Weingartner, H., Kaye, W., & Smalling, S. (1982). Determinants of memory failure in dementia. In S. Corkin, K. L. Davis, J. Growdon, E. Usdin, & R. J. Wurtman (Eds.), *Alzheimer's disease: A report of progress in research*. New York: Raven Press.

Wernicke, C. (1974). *Der aphasiche symptomen complex*. Breslau: Taschen.

Wertz, R. T. (1979). Review of word fluency measures (WF). In F. L. Darley (Ed.), *Evaluation of appraisal techniques in speech and language pathology*. Reading, MA: Addison-Wesley.

World Population Data Sheet (1986–1990). Washington, DC: Population Reference Bureau.

Xu, Y., Gong, Y. X., & Matthews, J. R. (1987). The Luria-Nebraska Neuropsychological Battery revised in China. *International Journal of Clinical Neuropsychology, 9*(3), 97–101.

Zagar, R., Arbit, J., Stuckey, M., & Wengel, W. W. (1984). Developmental analysis of the Wechsler Memory Scale. *Journal of Clinical Psychology, 40*, 1466–1473.

Author Index

Subject Index